BRAIN GLUCOSENSING:
PHYSIOLOGICAL IMPLICATIONS

NEUROLOGY - LABORATORY AND CLINICAL RESEARCH DEVELOPMENTS

Additional books in this series can be found on Nova's website under the Series tab.

Additional E-books in this series can be found on Nova's website under the E-book tab.

NEUROLOGY - LABORATORY AND
CLINICAL RESEARCH DEVELOPMENTS

BRAIN GLUCOSENSING: PHYSIOLOGICAL IMPLICATIONS

SERGIO POLAKOF

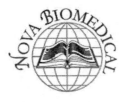

Nova Science Publishers, Inc.
New York

NOTICE TO THE READER

The Publisher has taken reasonable care in the preparation of this book, but makes no expressed or implied warranty of any kind and assumes no responsibility for any errors or omissions. No liability is assumed for incidental or consequential damages in connection with or arising out of information contained in this book. The Publisher shall not be liable for any special, consequential, or exemplary damages resulting, in whole or in part, from the readers' use of, or reliance upon, this material.

Independent verification should be sought for any data, advice or recommendations contained in this book. In addition, no responsibility is assumed by the publisher for any injury and/or damage to persons or property arising from any methods, products, instructions, ideas or otherwise contained in this publication.

This publication is designed to provide accurate and authoritative information with regard to the subject matter covered herein. It is sold with the clear understanding that the Publisher is not engaged in rendering legal or any other professional services. If legal or any other expert assistance is required, the services of a competent person should be sought. FROM A DECLARATION OF PARTICIPANTS JOINTLY ADOPTED BY A COMMITTEE OF THE AMERICAN BAR ASSOCIATION AND A COMMITTEE OF PUBLISHERS.

Library of Congress Cataloging-in-Publication Data

Polakof, Sergio.
 Brain glucosensing : physiological implications / author, Sergio Polakof.
     p. ; cm.
 Includes bibliographical references and index.
 ISBN 978-1-61761-334-0 (softcover)
 1. Glucose--Metabolism. 2. Brain. 3. Neurochemistry. 4. Homeostasis. 5.
Blood sugar. I. Title.
 [DNLM: 1. Brain--drug effects. 2. Glucose--physiology. 3.
Glucose--metabolism. QU 75]

 QP702.G560P65 2010
 572'.565--dc22
                              2010031170

Published by Nova Science Publishers, Inc. † *New York*

Contents

Preface

Glucose is an integral part of whole-body energy homeostasis and is tightly regulated by numerous endocrine, neuronal and behavioural systems, which ensure that glucose levels in the blood are maintained within a narrow physiological range.

The body continuously adapts its metabolism to keep blood glucose concentrations at a constant value. Glucose homeostasis in man and most other studied mammals is maintained by feedback designed to keep the blood glucose levels close to a set point characteristic for each species. Key to this homeostatic control is the existence of sensors located in different parts of the body that continuously monitor blood glucose variations. They respond to changes in glycemia by triggering hormonal secretion or activation of the autonomic nervous system to control glucose uptake, utilization or production and also to control energy expenditure and food intake.

The reliance of the brain on glucose to meet its energy demands suggests that, within the context of glucose homeostasis, brain glucosensing may predominate. Specialized neurons able to modulate their firing activity in response to changes in extracellular glucose levels were first demonstrated in the 1960s. These are glucose-excited (GE; previously called glucose responsive) neurons, which increase their firing rate when extracellular glucose concentrations elevate, or glucose-inhibited (GI; previously called glucose-sensitive) neurons, that are activated by a decrease in extracellular glucose concentration or by cellular glucoprivation. Both types of neurons are highly represented in brain regions involved in the control of energy homeostasis and food intake, suggesting that are able to receive inputs from blood nutrient and hormone levels, as well as from peripheral and central sensory systems, and use this information to generate the appropriate physiological response

Chapter I

Introduction

The central nervous system (CNS) has been identified as a key regulator of whole body homeostasis, playing a special role in regulating glucose metabolism. It is well known that the CNS senses and integrates information from a range of neural, hormonal and nutrient signals that are generated in response to the ingestion of food, which directly regulates glucose output by the liver and glucose uptake by peripheral tissues. It is also known that these homeostatic processes rely on the properly coordinated function of several peripheral organs, such as the liver, muscle, and adipose tissue, and the brain [1]. Moreover, it is clear now that this ability of the CNS to sense and respond to this information is impaired in overeating and obesity [2, 3]. On the other hand, selective CNS interventions in insulin resistance and diabetes animal models have been shown to ameliorate insulin resistance and hyperglycemia [2-5]. Obesity and the associated type 2 diabetes represent the major threats for human health in both developed and developing countries. Diabetes, which affects more than 170 million individuals world wide [6], is a disease characterized by impaired glucose homeostatic control. The difficulty in treating this disease stems in part from the relative lack of knowledge of the molecular mechanisms underlying the control of glucose homeostasis and metabolism [7]. Glucose is an important regulator signal that controls the secretion of hormones by various endocrine cells and activates neurons in the periphery and CNS. Since the brain rely mostly on glucose metabolism, requires that glycemia do not fall markedly below 5 mM, and thus glucosensing systems located in specific areas of the CNS are needed to control glucose homeostasis, feeding behaviour and energy storage and expenditure (Figure 1) [1].

Chapter II

Glucose Metabolism in the Brain

Glucose is transported into the brain cells through glucose transporters (GLUTs) independently of insulin. Although GLUTs have been found in all the brain cell types, GLUT1 is primarily located in the endothelial and astrocyte membranes, and GLUT3 are present on the neuronal cell membranes. It was shown that in response to insulin-induced hypoglycemia both GLUT1 and GLUT3 increase its presence in endothelial cells and neurons in order to improve glucose supply to the CNS [8]. After crossing the capillary endothelium, most glucose enters the astrocytes, which constitute the primary site of glucose metabolism in the brain and cover the 99% of the BBB basal lamina [9]. Once in the astrocyte, glucose is phosphorylated to glucose-6-phosphate (G6P) by hexokinases. Then, G6P can be metabolized by different pathways depending on the needs of the brain, that includes: i) conversion to pyruvate, ii) metabolization through the pentose phosphate pathway, and iii) storage as glycogen.

The conversion of G6P to pyruvate occurs in the cytoplasm of all the CNS cells directed by the key enzyme 6-phosphofructo-1-kinase (PFK-1), which increases pyruvate formation flux when ATP availability is low [10]. Pyruvate enters then the TCA cycle by pyruvate dehydrogenase (PDH) or a specific astrocyte pyruvate carboxylase (PC), and in the presence of oxygen is converted to acetyl-CoA which is combined with oxaloacetate in the formation of citrate [11]. Citrate is available as either an energy source to the cell's TCA cycle or as precursor to neurotransmitters synthesis (GABA, glutamate, α-ketoglutarate). Under anaerobic conditions, glycolytic flux increases and also the production of lactate. This metabolite is then exported by the cell (astrocytes) to the extracellular space and taken for other (neurons) through monocarboxylate transporters (MCTs) to be oxidized back to pyruvate and obtain ATP (see ANLSH section) [12].

The other pathway that the G6P can follow in the astrocyte is the pentose phosphate pathway, in which glucose is oxidized to ribulose-5-phosphate with an important production of NADPH. Glutathione is the main antioxidant in the brain [13], and the regeneration of the reduced glutathione requires NADPH as cofactor. Actually, the enhanced potential in pentose phosphate pathway is though to be related with a protecting function against oxidative injury in the brain during glucose deprivation [14].

Although under normal conditions very low levels of glycogen have been found in astrocytes, the role of this storage glucose product in brain energy homeostasis is though to be involved as fuel supplier during the short interval between activation of metabolism and increase delivery of glucose [15]. Glial glycogenolysis is linked to neuronal activity and the conversion of glycogen stores to glucose can be immediate during periods of hypoglycemia or increased neuronal metabolic demand, with vital importance to cell survival [16-18].

Chapter III

Sites of Glucosensing in the Brain

The first evidence suggesting the existence of neurons able to detect changes in glucose levels were provided by Claude Bernard, who lesioning the hypothalamus of dogs induced hyperglycemia [19]. Lately, it was proposed by Mayer the hypothesis of cells located in the hypothalamus specialized to monitor plasma glucose variations [20]. These cells could potentially "sense" the changes in glucose levels and translate them in electro-chemical signals that ultimately may regulate food intake. In 1954, Stellar proposed the "dual center" hypothesis of food intake, in which the ventromedial hypothalamus (VMH) is the "satiety center" and the lateral hypothalamus (LH) is the "feeding center" [21]. In the 1960s, for the first time, neurons able to modulate their firing activity in response to changes in extracellular glucose levels were identified by electrophysiological analysis of hypothalamic slices, [22, 23]. Those neurons were grouped, described and named by Oomura in 1964, and this nomenclature was used for 40 years. He named "glucose responsive" neurons to those neurons that increased their firing rate when ambient glucose levels rise. Conversely, "glucose sensitive" neurons were those inhibited by increasing glucose levels. More recently, Song and cols. (2001) proposed a new descriptive terminology for glucosensing neurons [24]. Thus, they named "glucose excited" (GE) neurons the glucose responsive neurons, and "glucose inhibited" (GI) neurons the glucose responsive neurons. Both types of neurons are widely distributed in the brain, although specially represented in hypothalamic nuclei and the brain stem, both regions involved in the control and regulation of energy homeostasis and food intake [7].

Within the hypothalamus, glucosensing neurons have been found in several nuclei, including VMN [22, 23, 25, 26], arcuate (Arc) [26-28], paraventricular (PVN) [29], suprachiasmatic [30, 31], and lateral (LH) [25, 32-37]. Besides the hypothalamus, other forebrain areas also contain glucosensing neurons, such as the septum [38], amygdale [39], stratium [40], and motor cortex [41]. Moreover, glucosensing neurons have been reported in a variety of other brain areas. Thus, within the hindbrain glucosensing neurons are present in substantia nigra [42-45], locus coeruleus [46], nucleus of the solitary tract (NTS) [36, 47, 48], dorsal vagal complex (DMNX) [49], and the area postrema (AP) [50]. Major glucosensing areas are shown in Figure 1.

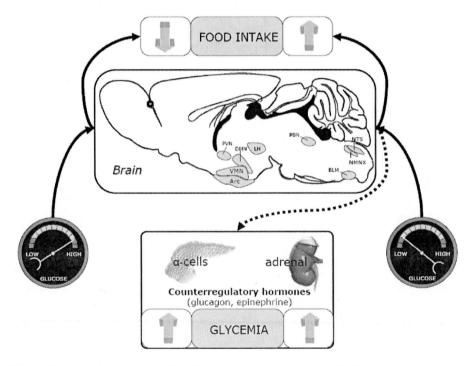

Figure 1. Brain sites of gluco-detection and schematic relationship between glucosensing brain areas and the control and regulation of food intake (solid arrows), and counterregulation to hypoglycemia (hatched arrows) during hypo- and hyperglycaemic episodes. Arc (arcuatus nucleus), VMN (ventromedial nucleus of the hypothalamus), DMN (dorsomedial nucleus of the hypothalamus), PVN (paraventricular nucleus of the hypothalamus), LH (lateral hypothalamus), PBN (parabranchial nucleus), BLM (basolateral medulla), NTS (nucleus of the solitary tract), DMNX (dorsal vagal complex).

Although some of the areas in which glucosensing areas are not related with the control and regulation of food intake and energy homeostasis, most of them present glucosensing neurons placed in specific areas involved in neuronendocrine and motor responses related with those functions [51]. Other evidence for the presence of glucosensing neurons has also been obtained by peripheral or central administrations of 2-deoxy-D-glucose (2-DG) or 5-thio-glucose (5-TG). The glucoprivation produced by these compounds induce metabolic or behavioural responses that allow identifying the activated neurons through electrophysiological or c-*fos*-like techniques. Neurons responding to glucoprivation were found in the Arc, VMN, PVN, LH, parabranchial nucleus (PBN), NTS, AP, DMNX, and the region of the basolateral medulla (BLM) [52-55].

Chapter IV

The Glucosensor Mechanism in the Brain

Unlike most neurons, glucosensing neurons use glucose as a signalling molecule to regulate their membrane potential and action potential frequency [56]. Although the mechanism by which glucosensing neurons detect changes in ambient glucose levels remains to be fully elucidated, GE neurons are currently considered as brain analogues of the pancreatic β-cells, whereas GI neurons have some similarities to α-cells [56].

4.1. Glucose-Excited Neurons

The current model describing the glucosensor mechanism in GE neurons has been inspired in the insulin-secreting mechanism in pancreatic β-cells. In the canonical β-cell model, glucose enters the cell *via* the GLUT2 glucose transporters, which permit rapid glucose uptake regardless of the extracellular sugar concentration [57]. At glucose levels <2.5 mM, little substrate is phosphorylated in β-cells [58], due to the low expression in these cells of high-affinity hexokinase (HK) isoforms, maintaining a low basal rate of insulin release. At glucose levels >2.5 mM, β-cells phosphorylate glucose *via* high-affinity glucokinase (GK) [59], that is not inhibited by G6P, and forms the basis of a proportional change in the cytoplasmic G6P concentration when extracellular glucose concentrations increase. This leads to a proportional increase in overall glycolytic flux and mitochondrial glucose oxidation. The crucial role of GK as the "gatekeeper" for metabolic signalling in β-cells is further illustrated by three observations [60]: i) β-cells with lower GK expression exhibit a lower glucose-induced insulin release than those with a higher expression [61]; ii) reduction of GK expression or functional enzyme activity is associated with an inadequate insulin-secretory response to glucose in patients with maturity onset diabetes of the young (MODY) [62]; and iii) targeted disruption of the GK gene in β-cells results in disturbed glucose-induced insulin release [63]. Tight coupling between glycolysis and mitochondrial oxidation has been considered to be crucial for more distal steps in the signal generation in β-cells [64]. The first and best characterized signal proceeds via K_{ATP} channels [65], since an acute rise in the extracellular glucose concentration from 1 to 10 mM glucose induces a dose-dependent increase in the ATP/ADP ratio [59]. This shift in adenine nucleotide pools is thought to stimulate insulin release *via* closure of K_{ATP} channels [65]. Intracellular ATP is indeed a negative allosteric regulator of the Kir6.2 pore-forming unit of these channels [66], whereas the concomitant decrease in ADP further contributes to this effect *via* the associated regulatory subunit, sulfonylurea receptor 1 (SUR1) [67]. The membrane depolarization that occurs upon closure of the K_{ATP} channels leads to the opening of L-type voltage-dependent calcium channels and induction of exocytosis [68] (Figure 2).

4.1.1. Glucose Transport

Because GE neurons increase their firing rate when ambient glucose levels rise, it was suggested that they may any share similarity with pancreatic β-cells [60, 69]. The presence of GLUT2 in hypothalamic nuclei where glucosensing neurons are present has been reported in several studies [7], although its involvement in glucose detection remains under debate. However, glucose transport does not seem to be the likely regulator of neuronal glucosensing [56]. The ubiquitous neuronal glucose transporter GLUT3 is fully saturated at most levels of brain glucose and is thereby unlikely to provide a gate-keeping function for glucosensing [70, 71].

Although GLUT2, the pancreatic β-cell glucose transporter, is expressed in most glucosensing neurons the fact that is also expressed in an equal number in non-glucosensing neurons suggest that is not either the critical determinant of the mechanism [56]. Other glucose transporters might be also participating in the glucosensing function. Insulin-dependent transporters GLUT4 were are expressed in both GE and GI neurons in addition to those mentioned above [70], although it is unlikely its involvement in the glucosensing function, since those neurons respond to changes in glucose levels in the absence of insulin [56]. In addition to GLUTs, the SGLT family of glucose transporters was also proposed as alternative to the metabolic glucosensing mechanism [72]. Studies carried out by O'Malley and cols (2006) demonstrated that the effects of both glucose and α-methylglucopyranoside are abolished by phloridzin (specific SGLT inhibitor) or by the removal of extracellular Na^+, suggesting that they were mediated predominantly by SGLTs [73]. These experiments indicate that the generation of ATP is not an essential prerequisite for glucosensing in many hypothalamic GE neurones, which instead can be non-metabolically excited by glucose via SGLTs [72]. However, although 25% of GE and 10% GI neurons express SGLT1, it remains to be elucidated which SGLT isoform(s) mediate these effects, since SGLT1-selective substrates activated a smaller proportion of GE neurones (37–45%) than SGLT1/3-non-selective sugars (67%). Since also SGLT3 transporter has been found in the brain [73, 74], it is possible that the SGLT1 was important but other SGLTs may also contribute to the non-metabolic pathway of glucosensing.

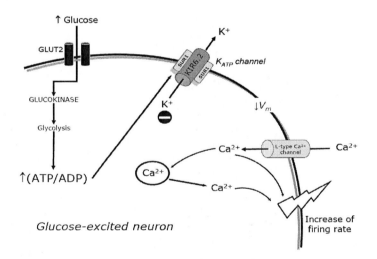

Figure 2. Hypothetical glucosensing mechanism in GE neurons. Glucose enters the GE neuron through GLUT 2, and is phosphorylated by GK, acting as the gatekeeper, and regulating the production of cytosolic ATP in a subcellular compartment. The ATP closes KATP channels in the plasma membrane, causing depolarization. In turn, this leads to Ca2+ influx through L-type Ca2+ channels, stimulating neurotransmitter release and increased action potential frequency. GLUT2 (glucose facilitative transporter type 2), KATP (ATP-sensitive inward rectified K+ channel), Kir6.2 (pore-forming subunit of KATP), SUR (sulfonylurea receptor).

4.1.2. Glucose Phosphorylation

Today is well recognized that GK is the primary regulator of glucosensing in most GE neurons [69, 70, 75]. The other HKs (mostly HK-I) are an unlikely regulator of glucosensing, since they are already saturated at physiological brain glucose concentrations and are inhibited by their reaction product, G6P [76]. The GK isoform expressed in the brain is the pancreatic [77], and is not inhibited by G6P [78], making suitable for glucosensing as in pancreatic β-cells. Although GK mRNA levels in the brain are low [75, 79], both GK immunoreactivity and activity have been found in the hypothalamus [76]. GK activity was described in the VMH and LH, where the changes in GK occur at the enzyme activity level rather than in transcriptional expression, suggesting that these modification should take place in short periods of time [80]. The low level of expression of this key enzyme is not surprising, since is only expressed in 20-40% of the total neural population, even in those areas known as glucosensors [77]. Despite this restricted protein distribution and low mRNA levels, GK gene expression highly correlates with the presence of glucosensing neurons in some brain areas. These include the PVN, VMN and Arc [69, 79, 81], as well as the NTS and AP [75]. The fact the GK is also expressed in other areas not previously tested as glucosensors, such as the lateral habenula, bed nucleus of the stria terminalis, inferior olive, retrochiasmatic and medial preoptic areas and thalamic posterior paraventricular, interpeduncular, oculomotor, and the anterior olfactory nuclei [79], remains to be elucidated. However, since glucose-induced alteration of neuronal activity correlates well with the presence of GK [75, 82], Levin *et al.* [77] have proposed that these areas could contain glucosensing neurons. The critical role of GK in GE neurons was further demonstrated when GE activity was decreased in neurons in which the enzyme was pharmacological inhibited [69, 70, 75, 83] or its mRNA interfered [84].

However, there are also many points that need to be clarified in order to elucidate the key role of GK as gatekeeper of the brain glucosensing system. The fact that an enzyme with high K_m as GK (about 8-10 mM) was able to regulate the glucosensing function at the range of brain glucose interstitial fluid remains to be fully investigated. It was proposed that GK activity could be modulated by interactions with other proteins like the GK regulatory protein (GKRP), as occurs in the liver and β-cells [85]. However, although the GKRP was found in the brain [86, 87], it is expressed only in 10% of GE neurons (and is not expressed in GI neurons) [70], making difficult such interaction. On the other hand, even when phosphofructo-2 kinase/fructose-

2,6-biphosphate is expressed also in the brain [88], possible interactions with GK remain to be tested.

4.1.3. Distal Sensing of Metabolic Signals

As in pancreatic β-cells [89], in GE neurons [90] the K_{ATP} channel is required to confer glucosensing capability. In the brain, K_{ATP} channel currents have been recorded in many regions, including substantia nigra [44], neocortex [91], hippocampus [92], and hypothalamus [93]. However, these K_{ATP} channels are expressed most abundantly in the hypothalamus, which is critically involved in the regulation of energy metabolism, controlling body weight and blood glucose levels [94].

The K_{ATP} channel is an octomeric functional unit composed of four pore-forming channels (Kir6.2) for K^+ and four binding sites for sulfonylureas [95]. The Kir6.2 pore-forming unit is a member of the inwardly rectifying K^+ channel family [96], while the sulfonylurea receptor (SUR) is a member of the ATP-binding cassette family. As with binding of ATP to the channel, occupation of the SUR inactivates the K_{ATP} channel and increases neuronal firing or transmitter release in GE neurons [51, 94]. In the brain both high glucose levels and the presence of sulfonylureas (or α-endosulfines [97]) lead to increased firing and/or transmitter release from GE neurons by their actions on the K_{ATP} channel. Interestingly, K_{ATP} channels are only present on GE neurons, but not in glia [98]. Kir6.2 and SUR1 are widely distributed in the brain, overlapping in numerous areas [98, 99], while SUR2 is more limited in its distribution to areas where GE neurons are present [99, 100]. More specifically, it was determined that SUR2, the low affinity form of the receptor, is mostly present in the cell bodies of the GE neurons, while SUR1, the high affinity form, is likely to be distributed on axon terminals [100], being the ratio Kir6.2 to SUR1/2 which determines the specificity of the channel to the metabolic changes [42]. This differential sensitivity was proposed as an explanation to the numerous differences found in the firing characteristics, conductances and sensitivities to glucose, sulfonylureas and ATP on many GE neurons [25, 51, 101]. In addition to these differences among GE neurons firing characteristics, some of them also show various subconductances of the K_{ATP} channel, which may vary depending upon the ambient conditions [102]. Another level of regulation is also the different inputs to a given neuron, since pre- and prosynaptics inputs may interplay, and the final output of this cell will be the sum of the direct effect of glucose on the cell body [45] and the axon

[103]. Neurons showing this behaviour include dopamine neurons in the substantia nigra [42, 98], norepinephrine neurons in the locus coeruleus [98], acetylcholine [104] and GABA [98] neurons in the striatum, and glutamate neurons in the motor cortex [103].

Although the K_{ATP} channel is an absolute requirement for glucosensing in GE neurons, since its deletion produces animals with no GE neurons in the VMH [90], it is unlikely to be the sole determinant of GE neuronal glucosensing, because it is present in many other neurons that have no apparent glucosensing capability [98]. In those neurons, it was proposed that the activation of K_{ATP} channels might play a protective role by hyperpolarizing the membrane as protection against the neurotoxic amounts of glutamate released when ATP levels fall during severe hypoglycemia and hypoxia [92].

However, there is also data suggesting that glucose could be detected by other mechanisms independent of GLUT2 [70], GK [105], and K_{ATP} [106]. It was proposed that the activation by glucose in some neurons GE could be dependent on the glucose-regulated activity of a transient response potential channel (TRP) [7, 106].

4.2. Glucose-Inhibited Neurons

The proximal mechanism of glucosensing in GI is similar to that described for GE neurons above. Thus, as in GE neurons, in GI neurons GK acts as the primary regulator of the glucosensor function [56]. GK mRNA is expressed in ~40% of GI neurons [70], and is critical in the proximal metabolic events responding to glucose [55, 70, 75]. Moreover, pharmacological inhibition of GK activity [55, 70, 75] as well as knockdown of GK mRNA [84] in VMH neurons *in vitro* abolishes the activity of GI neurons. Another important step in the proximal glucosensing mechanism in GI neurons is the glucose transport. It was shown that GI neurons express various types of glucose transporters, including GLUT2 [56], GLUT4 (~60%) [70] and SGLT1 (~10%) [70]. The mechanism linking a decrease in glucose concentration to increased firing activity is poorly known. Potential actors involved in this mechanism include the Na^+-K^+-ATPase pump [25, 107], ATP-activated K^+ channel [101], and a chloride channel [105, 108] (Figure 3).

The involvement of the Na^+-K^+-ATPase was originally proposed by Oomura et al. [107], which using oubain (Na^+-K^+-ATPase blocker) suggested that glucose could stimulate this pump, inhibiting the cell. However, the effect of this blocker was reversible and probably due to indirect phenomena [109], and the contribution of the Na^+-K^+-ATPase to the glucosensing mechanism in GI neurons remain to be elucidated to this day.

From *in vitro* recordings of currents in mediobasal hypothalamic neurons Song and cols. [24] have put forward the hypothesis that relates the inhibitory effect of glucose in GI neurons with the activation of post-synaptic Cl^- channels, probably belonging to the CFTR family. More recently, Fioramonti et al. [110] found in Arc GI neurons that increasing glucose levels activated a membrane current depending on the Cl^- intracellular concentration. Further pharmacological support to this idea was obtained using gemfibrozil (a CFTR Cl^- channel blocker), that when added to the media make GI neurons unable to respond to glucose stimulus [110]. However, the fact the gemfibrozil itself is able to hyperpolarize the cell and that those studies were carried out with low $[Cl^-]$ solutions make difficult to interpret these data.

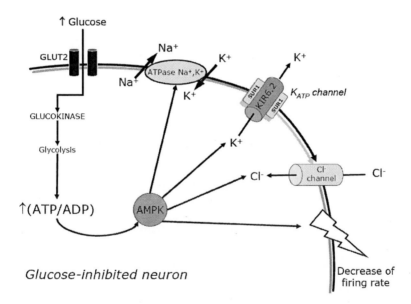

Figure 3. Hypothetical glucosensing mechanism in GI neurons. In GI neurons, GK may act as the gatekeeper. A falling glucose results in an increase in the AMP:ATP ratio, activating AMPK. AMPK may act on chloride channels, KATP channels and/or Na+/K+ ATPase, leading to neuronal depolarization and neurotransmitter release and/or decreased action potential frequency. GLUT2 (glucose facilitative transporter type 2), KATP (ATP-sensitive inward rectified K+ channel), Kir6.2 (pore-forming subunit of KATP), SUR (sulfonylurea receptor), AMPK (AMP-activated protein kinase).

On the other hand, the measurement of membrane current-voltage relationship using high [Cl⁻] pipette solutions shows that glucose activates a current selective for K^+ ions [111]. The fact the increased glucose concentration in the medium triggers large post-synaptic K^+ currents suggest that at least in orexin neurons these are the final effectors [109].

Chapter V

Lactate as Metabolic Coupling between Astrocytes and Glucosensing Neurons

Because of the symbiotic relationship between astrocytes and neurons proposed in the astrocyte-neuron lactate shuttle hypothesis (ANLSH) [112], astrocyte-derived lactate was proposed as regulator of activity in glucosensing neurons [56] (Figure 4). Astrocytes take up and store transported glucose as glycogen, releasing lactate into the extracellular space [112]. Astrocyte glycogen stores can sustain neuron metabolism during short-term glucoprivic (low glucose availability) conditions [113]. Lactate is transported into glucosensing neurons from the extracellular space by type 1 monocarboxylate transporters (MCT-2), where it is converted by lactate dehydrogenase (LDH) to pyruvate, which is then oxidized in mitochondria to provide ATP [70, 114].

The specific kinetics of the MCTs and the isoforms of LDH on astrocytes (MCT-1, LDH-5) vs neurons (MCT-2, LDH-1) suggest that astrocytes are a lactate "source" while neurons are a lactate "sink" [12]. Therefore, in most neurons, astrocyte-derived lactate can be converted to pyruvate to provide a ready source of ATP production [51]. Thus, in glucosensing neurons glucose can act as either a direct (glycolysis in neurons) or indirect (astrocyte-derived lactate) source of neuronal substrate to produce ATP [51]. Further support to this hypothesis was found in the results of Ainscow and cols., who reported that hypothalamic glia (but not neurons) respond to a rise in extracellular glucose with a large increase in glycolytic ATP production, which would be expected to lead to glial release of lactate [115, 116]. More recently, it was also demonstrated that lactate has excitatory actions and could be involved in glucose metabolism on GE neurons of the hypothalamus, but not on non-glucosensing neurons [105, 117]. In contrast, pharmacological disruption of metabolic coupling between neurons and astrocytes *in vivo* prevented glucose-induced c-*fos* activation in Arc neurons of the hypothalamus [118]. In the brain stem, lactate is sensed as a metabolic signal that can regulate the activation of GE neurons in the AP and NTS, as detected by c-*fos* labelling studies, and blocking MCTs by injection in the fourth ventricle, which leads to elevations in blood glucose levels [119-121]. Moreover, it was recently demonstrated that DMNX neuronal utilization of both lactate and glucose may be enhanced in response to local lactate abundance, alone or relative to glucose scarcity [122].

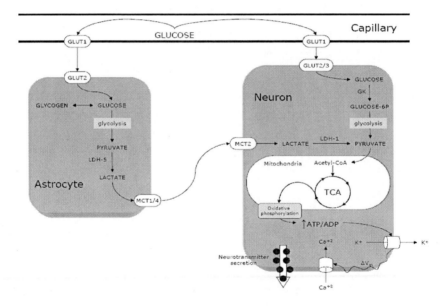

Figure 4. Relationship between brain capillary, astrocyte, and neuron and glucose metabolism. Glucose is transported across the microvessel by GLUT1 and enters either the astrocyte by GLUT2 transport or the extracellular space, where it is transported into a GE neuron by GLUT2/3. This leads to increased lactacte production and transfer to neurons through the monocarboxylate transporters MCT1/4 and MCT2 and a consequent augmentation in pyruvate formation in neurons and increased ATP production. In GE neurons, the increase in in ATP-to-ADP ratio leads to activation of the KATP channels and plasma membrane depolarization, and thus increase in neuronal firing activity and neurotransmitters release. GLUT2 (glucose facilitative transporter type 2), GK (glucokinase), LDH (lactic dehydrogenase), MCT (monocarboxylate transporter).

However, despite this ability to transport and use the astrocyte-derived lactate as a metabolic signalling molecule, it was also demonstrated that glucosensing neurons are able to respond to glucose in the complete absence of this metabolite [70, 75]. The fact that glucosensing and non-glucosensing neurons appear to express both MCT and LDH in equivalent abundance make it likely that astrocyte-derived lactate is more often used as an alternative substrate to support neuronal metabolism than as a signalling molecule to regulate activity [70, 75, 123].

Chapter VI

Network of Hypothalamic Glucosensing Neurons

6.1. Neurons of the Arcuatus Nucleus

The actions exerted by NPY (stimulation of appetite and suppression of energy expenditure) and POMC (inhibition of feeding and stimulation of energy expenditure) neurons are thought to be mediated by the projections from Arc of these neurons to several CNS regions that control appetite and metabolism [124]. A crucial characteristic of this system is that the activity of NPY and POMC neurons is oppositely regulated by signals of body energy status, avoiding contradictory influences. If glucose is able to excite POMC neurons and inhibit NPY neurons remains to be elucidated, although there are many studies supporting this model. Data from NPY glucosensing neurons was obtained from indirect activity determinations, such as changes in intracellular calcium concentration. In this sense, data from Muroya et al. [27] suggest that Arc NPY neurons could be directly inhibited by glucose. On the other hand, data from Arc POMC glucosensing neurons are contradictory and likely species-dependent. While in mouse 80% of POMC neurons are excited by glucose [125], in rat Wang et al. [83] failed to detect glucose-excited neurons in Arc preparations. More studies are needed to clarify if this discrepancy is an indicative of species differences or is due to different populations of POMC neurons within the Arc.

6.2. Neurons of the Ventromedial Nucleus

Unlike other hypothalamic nuclei, no endogenous neurochemical markers are known in the VMN neurons, making difficult to relate glucosensing neurons with putative functions and connections. In this sense, RT-PCR studies have shown that GE neurons of this nucleus are GABAergic [70, 90]. However, no information about the possible targets or connections with these neurons is available, and then further studies in this nucleus are needed to understand better the physiological implication of VMN glucosensing neurons.

6.3. Neurons of the Lateral Nucleus

The first evidence that LH orexin neurons might be GI neurons was obtained from *in vivo* experiments in which systemic hypoglycemia activates orexin neurons [126, 127]. However, initially orexin-A expression was not found in glucosensing neurons of this hypothalamic region [128]. In contrast, another study published at the same time show that some of the orexin cells of the LH respond to extracellular glucose changes [129]. Further confirmation of these results was found later in the hyperpolarizing ability of glucose on 80-100 % of LH-orexin neurons in the physiological glucose range (0.2-5 mM) [130, 131]. These data demonstrate that glucose is able to inhibit LH-orexin neurons, and suggest that these neurons could be stimulated when glucose levels fall [132]. Actually, the fact the mice whose orexin neurons were specifically destroyed failed to respond to fasting, supports the involvement of orexin-LH glucosensing neurons in energy homeostasis and food intake regulation [130, 133]. In this sense, direct excitatory actions of orexins on appetite-promoting Arc NPY/AgRP neurons [134] and indirect inhibitory effects of orexins on anorexigenic Arc POMC neurons [135] have been proposed to contribute to appetite-stimulating effects of orexins administration [136]. However, the net effect of orexins on energy balance seems to be negative, since loss of orexin neurons causes obesity and diminished energy expenditure and locomotor activity [137].

Besides orexin neurons, there are also melanin-concentrating hormone (MCH) neurons in the LH. However, MCH neurons seem to have opposite roles to those of orexin neurons, since MCH knock-out mice exhibited increased metabolic rate and reduced body weight [138]. Recent results from Burdakov et al. [131] showed that in the LH 80% of MCH neurons are directly excited by glucose within the physiological range. Accordingly with the functions exerted by MCH, it was suggested that glucose-induced excitation of MCH neurons may suppress energy expenditure [132].

Chapter VII

The Mechanisms Underlying Glucosensing During Hypoglycemia

Hypoglycemia results in reduced brain cell energy production and an imbalance in neurotransmitters. Mild hypoglycemia leads to brain cell dysfunction by causing neuroexcitation and elevations in intracellular calcium, sodium and potassium levels. Severe hypoglycemia leads to brain-cell death. Hypoglycemia is especially important in type 1 diabetes mellitus (T1DM), and is still the most frequent and dangerous side-effect of insulin therapy. Despite the introduction of insulin analogues and improved delivery systems, hypoglycemia remains as the main limitation to achieving near-normal glucose control in T1DM patients [139]. Then, understanding the mechanisms of glucose metabolism and utilization within the CNS will allow the exploration of metabolic interventions designed to minimize or prevent damage to brain cells [10]. In this sense, is critical to focus the attention in the ability of the CNS to detect hypoglycemia and protect itself from this it.

Under normal physiological conditions, plasma glucose levels are about 4-10 mM, while interstitial brain glucose levels are maintained about 20-30% of those in plasma, between 1-3 mM [140, 141]. Moreover, there are also considerable regional differences [141-144] that become accentuated when plasma glucose levels fall. These differences in regional glucose levels have important implications for cerebral metabolism, glucosensing, but specially for selective vulnerability during states of hypoglycemia [51]. When plasma glucose levels approach 3.6–3.8 mM, clinical signs such as nervousness, tremors, cardiac palpitations, and weakness have been observed in human, rat, mice, rabbit, cat, dog, and monkey [11]. When plasma glucose levels fall below 1 mM, seizure activity, severe brain damage, coma, and death can occur as a result of neuronal dysfunction and cell death [11, 145]. Globally, hypoglycemia stimulates glucosensors, initiating the compensatory mechanisms that increase plasma glucose concentration, glucose delivery and uptake by the brain. In order to prevent the clinical signs of hypoglycemia cited above and to minimize brain cell injury, both central and systemic adaptative changes must be rapid and effective counteracting plasma glucose fall.

7.1. Systemic Mechanism Against Hypoglycemia

As stated above, when blood glucose levels fall below ~5 mM a rapid counterregulatory response to restore normoglycemia is initiated. This involves a first decrease in insulin secretion and a concomitant increase in glucagon concentration and secretion that should restore normoglycemia through stimulation of glycogenolysis and gluconeogenesis in the liver, which is also activated directly *via* the autonomic nervous system [146-148]. If plasma glucose levels remain low, then a second mechanism is triggered. The VMH initiates the release of epinephrine and norepinephrine from adrenal glands [149]. If hypoglycemia persists for hours, a third mechanism initiates the secretion of cortisol and growth hormone. It is likely that both brain and hepatic portal glucosensors participate in this response [150, 151].

7.2. Metabolic Central Counterregulation

During hypoglycemia several changes take place in the brain in order to increase glucose delivery to the CNS. Thus, GLUTs increase in the brain the cerebral blood flow shifts to enhance glucose uptake [152]. Actually, during hypoglycemic episodes, GLUT1 translocate from intracellular stores to the plasmatic membrane (up to 50%) in order to increase glucose extraction from the blood [153]. Moreover, GLUT3 in neurons increase in number, enhancing glucose uptake from the extracellular fluid [11]. When these mechanisms are unable to maintain the glucose supply and uptake remain ineffective, then the local metabolism is modified in order to keep the ATP levels high. Thus, an increase towards pyruvate and lactate production takes place in the brain glycolytic pathway [154]. Local lactate production is usually effective maintaining the energy supply to the brain during the initial stages of chronic hypoglycemia [155]. In addition, glycogen stores in the astrocytes are depleted in order to provide additional energy substrates [10].

7.3. Sites of Detection of Hypoglycemia

The sites of central hypoglycemia detection are widely distributed through the brain and can be activated either by hypoglycemia or by peripheral or central glucoprivation [7] (Figure 1). The role of central glucosensors areas in hypoglycemia detection has been classically evidenced by two different approaches: i) intracarotid glucose infusion, that blocks hypoglycemia-induced secretion of counterregulatory hormones and endogenous glucose production [151, 156]; ii) intracerebroventroicular injection of glucoprivic agents like 2-deoxy-glucose (2-DG), which stimulates glucagon and catecholamine secretion and endogenous glucose production to induce hyperglycemia [157].

Evidence that hypothalamic areas are involved in the detection of hypoglycemia have been elucidated after the injection of 2-DG directly into the VMH, inducing glucagon secretion [157]. Inversely, hypoglycemia-induced glucagon secretion can be suppressed by injecting glucose in that same hypothalamic area [158]. The same authors have also demonstrated that after lesioning the VMH the counterregulatory response is attenuated by 75% [159]. Other factors involved in the regulation of the counterregulatory response against hypoglycemia as corticotrophin-releasing factors (CRF) and urocortins are able to either increase or suppress respectively hypoglycemia-induced counterregulation, modulating directly the firing rate of VMH glucosensing neurons [160, 161]. Besides VMH, other hypothalamic areas are also involved in this function. Thus, in the LH the infusion of glucoprivic 2-DG also stimu http://notifier.avira.com/stats.php?id_not=380&url=https %3A%2F%2Favira.cleverbridge.com%2F30%2Fcookie%3Fx-origin%3 Dnotifier% 26x-notifier%3D30days_EN%26expiry%3D40% 26redirectto% 3Dhttp%253A%252F%252Fwww.avira.de%252Fen%252Fproducts%252Ftest _avira_premium_security_suite.htmllates activity in the adrenal nerve, but inhibits sympathetic activation of brown adipose tissue [162]. In the DMH, 2-DG also inhibits adrenal nerve activity [163].

There is also evidence that other brain areas are involved in the detection of hypoglycemia and counterregulation. For instance, caudal brain stem norepinephrine and epinephrine neurons that project to the spinal cord are necessary for the full expression of this response [164]. Other evidence was obtained from different approaches, such as the obstruction of the cerebral aqueduct that communicates the third and fourth ventricles. Under these conditions, the 5-TG-induced glucoregulatory response can be only achieved when the administration is made in the fourth but not in the third ventricle [165]. Interestingly, 5-TG injection that fails to induce a glucoregulatory response in the hypothalamus [166], when is administered in the NTS and the basomedullary regions containing catecholaminergic neurons (that project to the hypothalamus), induces a strong response [164, 167]. Moreover, immunostaining techniques have demonstrated that the preserved response against intraperitoneal injection of 2-DG in decerebrated rats [168] involves the activation of neurons present in the NTS, DMNX and the basolateral medulla [169].

7.4. Counterregulation to Hypoglycemia in T1DM: Why Glucosensor Mechanisms Fail?

As stated above, in health a fall in plasma glucose levels is rapidly detected and a sequence of counterregulatory responses is triggered in order to recover normoglycemia as soon as possible. However, in T1DM patients these compensatory systems are disrupted at every level. One of them is the defect in glucagon secretion, which made T1DM patients very reliant on the sympathoadrenal response to hypoglycemia to restore normoglycemia. However, this response is also impaired over time in T1DM [170], and the major reason for the development of this defect is thought to be the experience of hypoglycemia itself. Thus, the frequent hypoglycemia experienced by insulin intensive therapy in T1DM patients lower the glucose level at which hormonal counterregulation is initiated [171], and then episodes of precedent hypoglycemia lead to suppressed epinephrine responses to a subsequent episode of hypoglycemia [172]. Data from rodent studies suggest that this defect in the glucorregulatory response arises through changes in specific glucosensing brain regions, such as the VMH [173]. Recurrent hypoglycemia has been shown to suppress the counterregulatory response to 2-DG infusions into the VMH, and even the glucose levels at which the first activation of glucosensor neurons take place is lower in those animals experiencing prior recurrent hypoglycemia [174]. Other experimental evidence supporting this contention include the restoration of normal counterregulatory response to subsequent hypoglycemia in rats suffering recurrent hypoglycemic episodes and in which 5-AMP-activated protein kinase (AMPK) activation and K_{ATP} opening channel in the VMH occurred [175]. In order to explain this model, Mc Crimmon (2008) have suggested that the balance between GE and GI neurons activity could be altered by recurrent hypoglycemia and that this unbalance might be responsible of this lower glucose level at which the counterregulatory response against hypoglycemia is started [172].

7.5. Glucosensing Markers Involved in the Counterregulatory Response to Hypoglycemia

The role of glucosensing neurons containing GLUT2 transporters and involved in the counterregulatory response against hypoglycemia has been demonstrated with transgenic mice [176]. In these mice, the absence of this glucose carrier leads to an exaggerated glucagon secretion due to an increased autonomic tone. Moreover, administration of 2-DG (central or peripherally) failed to stimulate glucagon secretion. Later studies showed that the GLUT2-dependent glucosensors involved in the counterregulatory response to hypoglycemia are associated rather to brain stem structures, such as NTS and DMNX, than hypothalamic areas, like the VMH [177]. More specifically, in GLUT2 defective mice the counterregulatory response against hypoglycemia was only restored when the glucose carrier was expressed in glial cells in the brain stem, reinforcing the model of glucosensing units composed by neurons and astrocytes [177]. Accordingly with the ANLSH, the basis of this unit may be the metabolic coupling between neurons and astrocytes [12].

The involvement of GK in the counterregulatory response against hypoglycemia has been assessed through intracerebroventricular administration of inhibitors as alloxan. Alloxan increases mRNA levels of GK in the hypothalamus, inhibiting the hyperglycemic response induced by glucoprivation. However, the effect is transient and when GK expression levels are restored, the response is normalized [178, 179]. More recently, this concept was reviewed, with more emphasis on GK activity instead gene expression as key regulator of the response [180]. When a GK activator was injected into the VMH *in vivo*, the increases in GK activity resulted in reduced epinephrine, norepinephrine and glucagon responses to the insulin-induced hypoglycemia. However, when GK activity or gene expression were reduced as consequence of alloxan injection in the VMH, the effect was lesser and more selective, increasing primarily the epinephrine response to insulin-induced hypoglycemia [180]. The authors explained the last results based on the low levels of GK expression in the normal brain [75, 76] and the low affinity of GK in relationship to the levels of brain glucose, particularly during insulin-induced hypoglycemia [181], which can make GK more adequate as glucosensing regulator within the normal physiological range. However, during severe hypoglycemia, it seems that GK may play a less prominent role in stimulating the counterregulatory response than enzymes such as AMPK, which are highly sensitive to low levels of ATP.

Some of the evidence that involve the K_{ATP} in the counterregulation against hypoglycemia has been obtained from null mice. Thus, Kir6.2 null mice show markedly delayed recovery from insulin-induced systemic hypoglycemia, suggesting impaired secretion of counterregulatory hormones such as glucagon and catecholamines. However, while epinephrine secretion in response to insulin-induced hypoglycemia in Kir6.2 null mice is similar to that in wild-type *in vivo*, glucagon secretion is markedly reduced [90]. Moreover, other characteristics of the glucosensing neurons were altered in these mice, such as the lack of spontaneous discharge rate in VMH neurons in response to glucose (as occur in the wild-type). These findings show that Kir6.2-containing K_{ATP} channels are required for glucose responsiveness of glucosensing neurons in the VMH. Studies of intracerebroventricular injections also demonstrate the involvement of these channels in the recognition of hypoglycemia, since K_{ATP} inhibitors injected in the VMH are able to block the counterregulatory response to a hypoglycemic clamp or glucose deprivation (5-TG administration) [182]. In contrast, when K_{ATP} are activated specifically in the same area the counterregulatory hormonal response against single or recurrent hypoglycemia results amplified [183].

Recent evidence has emerged to suggest that AMPK may play a role in the sensing of hypoglycemia within the VMH. AMPK is activated during cellular energy depletion and acts to suppress ATP-consuming pathways and to activate ATP-generating pathways, which has led to it being called an intracellular "fuel gauge " [184]. Hypothalamic AMPK has also been implicated in the regulation of counterregulatory response to acute hypoglycemia [145, 175, 185], and 5-aminoimidazole-4-carboxamide-1-β-D-ribofuranoside (AICAR), a pharmacological activator of AMPK, mimics the effect of low glucose to stimulate neuronal activity in VMH glucose-inhibited neurons [186]. On the contrary, blocking hypothalamic AMPK with compound C or by expressing a dominant negative form of the kinase strongly reduced counterregulation to insulin-induced hypoglycemia [185]. Recently, the involvement of AMPK in this process was confirmed utilizing shRNAs. In this study [187], VMH AMPK down-regulation resulted in suppressed glucagon (60%) and epinephrine (40%) responses to acute hypoglycemia when compared with controls. In addition, animals with VMH AMPK down-regulation also required more exogenous glucose to maintain the hypoglycemia plateau and showed significant reductions in endogenous glucose production and whole-body glucose uptake.

Chapter VIII

Brain Glucosensing and the Regulation of Food Intake and Energy Expenditure

Food intake is the most important source of glucose and this led Mayer to propose in 1953 the existence of a feedback loop in which glucose oxidation was sensed, and this information utilized to regulate food intake [20]. After the *glucostatic hypothesis* of Mayer many studies have evaluated glucose regulation of food intake.

In rodents [188-190] and humans [191] meal initiation was usually linked to a rise in blood glucose levels which follows directly after a small dip (about 10%, ~0.5 mM) in glucose levels (Figure 1). Since this variation in blood glucose levels is very small, it was proposed that glucosensing neurons should be able to detect especially little changes in glucose to be involved in the meal initiation process. Usually, brain glucose levels represent about 20-30% of those in plasma [144], and then glucosensing neurons should be able to detect variation of 0.1-0.15 mM, corresponding to the 0.5 mM dip in blood glucose levels associated with meal initiation. Actually, it was demonstrated that some hypothalamic neurons are able to respond within this range, being its involvement in meal initiation a real possibility [25]. However, these data should be interpreted carefully, because not all meals are preceded by such dips [188, 189] and then the involvement of glucosensing neurons could just explain one of the possible existing mechanisms. Recently, the involvement of glucosensing neurons of the hypothalamus (VMH) as mediator of spontaneous and glucoprivic feeding was assessed [192]. Although changes in both plasma and VMH glucose levels were associated with spontaneous meals, the authors showed that was the low glucose rather than the changing levels what stimulates the glucoprivic meals. Thus, although VMH glucosensing does not appear to be involved in either spontaneous feeding or long-term body-weight regulation, it does participate in glucoprivic feeding [192]. In this sense, glucoprivation has been traditionally used to study the effect of glucose on meal initiation in many studies [165, 167, 168, 193]. Experimentally, induction of cellular glucoprivation by administration of 2-DG either peripherally [194] or centrally [195, 196] induces food intake. More precisely, the main glucosensing area in which local glucoprivation was effectively a food intake induced was the hindbrain, since glucoprivation of other brain areas, such as the LH or VMH [196] failed to elicit this response. Supporting these results, direct glucoprivation (5-TG injection) into the BLM, DMNX and NTS was able to stimulate food intake in rodents [167]. However, since the intracellular glucopenia produced by these agents stimulates both food intake and a counterregulatory neuroendocrine response [193, 197], it was suggested that the feeding response evoked by glucoprivation is not equivalent to that observed during diurnal normal ingestive behaviour [51]. Alternatively, fasting and insulin-induced hypoglycemia have been used to stimulate feeding. Blood glucose does drop during night-time fasting and rats will eat more rapidly when re-exposed to food after such a fast: the lower the level of glucose reached during fasting, the higher the rate of refeeding when food is made readily available [198]. However, the numerous metabolic events that accompany fasting, such as a precipitous drop in plasma leptin [199], also a trigger of meal initiation [200], prevent to interpret these data so easily. From these data seems to be clear that glucose acts as a physiologic regulator of ingestion, and it was proposed then that the pathways mediating glucoprivic feeding may be separate from those modulating the physiologic control of ingestion [51]. In fact, there are many physiological conditions in which glucoprivic feeding is rendered defective and feeding responses to other physiologic modulators of food intake such as NPY, leptin, and cholecystokinin are preserved [90, 201, 202]. As part of this dissociation, also anatomical differences were noticed, since the peptides and neurotransmitters mentioned above intrinsic to the hypothalamus and other forebrain areas are considered to be physiological regulators of ingestive behaviour [203-206], while glucoprivic feeding appears to be integrated and initiated primarily within hindbrain sites [164, 165, 167, 168]. However, numerous studies also demonstrated that neurons mediating glucoprivic feeding are integrated in normal diurnal food intake [90, 164, 203, 207], suggesting that are separate but highly overlapping systems mediating glucoprivic and normal diurnal ingestive behaviour [51].

8.1. Glucosensing Markers Involved in The Control of Food Intake and Energy Expenditure

Most of the results that suggest an involvement of central GLUT2 in the regulation of food intake have been obtained from experiments with GLUT2 antisense oligonucleotides [7]. In GLUT2 null mice both central and peripheral glucose injections are unable to reduce food intake [208], suggesting that a defect in central glucosensing must exist. Moreover, in null mice for GLUT2 2-DG is no longer recognized as feeding regulator [209].

Other components of the glucosensor system have also studied (mostly through pharmacological approaches) in order to elucidate their involvement in glucose detection and food intake, such as GK. Thus, Ritter and Strang (1982) [210] showed that intracerebroventricular injections of the GK inhibitor alloxan reduce food intake in rats. However, paradoxical effects were also found when the drug was administered at higher doses, since both GK activity and expression were noticed in the hypothalamus. In addition, the feeding response to peripheral 2-DG administration was transiently enhanced. The explanation proposed was that higher GK activity and mRNA levels could probably increase glucose metabolism and ATP levels, preventing the initiation of the feeding process [178].

Little information is available regarding the involvement of the central K_{ATP} channels in food intake regulation. Utilizing null mice for Kir6.2 gene it was demonstrated that the increased feeding response to peripheral 2-DG administration was reduced in mice lacking this K_{ATP} channel subunit [90]. More recently, it was demonstrated that changes in Kir6.2 gene expression and location may alter the activity of neurons controlling the food intake response, such as NPY and AgRP neurons, where Kir6.2 was co-localized [211].

In recent years, AMPK has emerged as a sensor for nutrients, specially glucose, in the hypothalamus [212, 213] and its role in appetite regulation has been thoroughly investigated [214]. AMPK is widely expressed throughout the brain, including several areas controlling food intake and neuroendocrine function such as the hypothalamus and the hindbrain [215]. Hypothalamic AMPK is influenced by energy intake and availability, as well as by several orexigenic and anorexigenic signals [216]. Leptin decreases hypothalamic AMPK activity in Arc and PVN [216, 217] leading to reduced appetite with consequent reduction of body weight. Furthermore, inhibition of hypothalamic AMPK is necessary for leptin's effects on food intake and body weight, as constitutively active AMPK blocks these effects. More recently it was demonstrated that AMPK regulates the inhibitory effect of leptin on the electrical activity of GI neurons [218]. Ghrelin, a circulating growth hormone-releasing and appetite-inducing brain-gut peptide [219], stimulates hypothalamic AMPK following either intraperitoneal or intracerebroventricular injection [220], suggesting that AMPK activation might be part of its orexigenic effect. Both exogenous and endogenous cannabinoids stimulate appetite in the hypothalamus *via* cannabinoid receptor type 1 [221]. Furthermore, cannabinoids stimulate AMPK activity in the hypothalamus, which could explain their central orexigenic effects [220]. Adiponectin enhances AMPK activity in the Arc after re-feeding, stimulates food intake and decreases energy expenditure [222]. Conversely, adiponectin-deficient mice showed decreased AMPK phosphorylation in the Arc, decreased food intake, and increased energy expenditure. Under fasting conditions, high adiponectin levels would stimulate AMPK and food intake and would decrease energy expenditure. After re-feeding adiponectin levels would fall with a consequent decrease in AMPK activity and food intake and an increase in energy expenditure. Nevertheless, recent studies showed that, in contrast to the situation in pancreatic β-cells [223, 224], the K_{ATP} channel-independent effects of glucose on GE neurons were unlikely to involve changes in AMPK activity [218]. Moreover, more recently it was demonstrated with AMPKα2 knock-outs that the regulation of food intake is independent of glucosensing in either POMC or AgRP neurons [225]. In contrast to GE neurons, changes in AMPK activity are likely to mediate the effects of glucose on BMN GI neurons, a proportion of which express NPY [218]. Thus, it has been proposed that AMPK may be involved in the activation of BMN GI neurons at low glucose concentrations, since glucose uptake and metabolism would fall, and the resulting increase in the AMP:ATP ratio would then lead to an activation of AMPK [226]. It is possible that AMPK may then act to directly phosphorylate and inactivate plasma membrane Cl⁻ and possibly other ion channels [24], leading to cell depolarization, and activation of the neurons. Enhanced release of the orexigenic peptide NPY from some GI neurones could act *via* a series of 'second-order' neurons to regulate cerebral cortex and autonomic preganglionic neurones involved in controlling feeding behaviour [227].

Chapter IX

Glucosensing Neurons as Metabolic Sensors

The fact that glucosensing neurons are located in brain areas specifically involved in the regulation of food intake and energy homeostasis, such as some hypothalamic and brain stem nuclei, suggest that these neurons do more than just sense glucose [228]. Then, besides glucose, glucosensing neurons respond to many other metabolites, including lactate, ketone bodies and free fatty acids [33, 55, 69, 122, 229, 230]. These specialized neurons act not only as glucosensors but also as metabolic sensors, since receive a host of other metabolic, hormonal and neural signals. Glucosensing neurons also express receptors for and respond to peripheral hormones that convey signals relating to fat stores such as leptin [231] and insulin [83]. Both leptin [231] and insulin [232] decrease action potential frequency in GE neurons at high glucose concentrations. Long-chain acyl-CoA also activates the K_{ATP} channel [233] as well as inhibits GK activity [234]. Thus, glucosensing neurons have been re-defined by Levin [56] as *"metabolic sensors"* in which a variety of metabolic, hormonal, transmitter, and peptide signals related to metabolic status are summated at the level of the membrane potential to alter neuronal activity (Figure 5).

Anabolic Arc NPY neurons and catabolic POMC neurons are examples of these metabolic sensors, because they are equipped and locate to play a key role in the regulation of energy homeostasis [56]. Arc NPY neurons project to the PVN, which is linked to both neuroendocrine and autonomic effect pathways [235], and restriction of energy intake [236] and glucoprivation

[237] increase NPY expression selectively on those neurons. Arc POMC neurons have similar projection fields to Arc NPY neurons [227, 238].

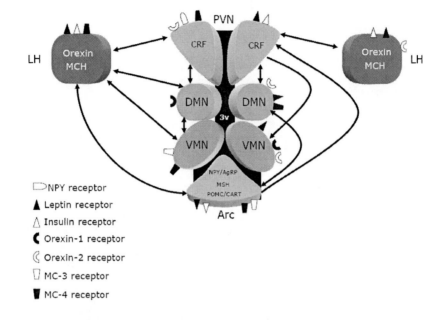

NPY receptor
Leptin receptor
Insulin receptor
Orexin-1 receptor
Orexin-2 receptor
MC-3 receptor
MC-4 receptor

Figure 5. Hypothalamic network of glucosensing cells. The putative interconnecting synaptic contacts between hypothalamic nuclei are indicated with arrows. Soft gray shading represent sites with GE neurons, while strong gray shadow represent sytes with GI neurons. Receptors to different peptides and hormones are also represented. Arc (arcuatus nucleus), VMN (ventromedial nucleus of the hypothalamus), DMN (dorsomedial nucleus of the hypothalamus), PVN (paraventricular nucleus of the hypothalamus), LH (lateral hypothalamus), CRF (corticotropin-releasing factor), MCH (melanin-concentrating hormone), MSH (melanocyte-stimulating hormone), NPY (neuropeptide Y), AgRP (agouti related protein), POMC (pro-opiomelanocortin), CART (cocaine- and amphetamine-regulated transcript).

However, these POMC neurons produce α-MSH, which interacts with catabolic melanocortin receptors [239], decreasing food intake [240]. On the other hand, NPY neurons have been described as GI, and POMC neurons are GE [27, 125]. Both types of neurons express Kir6.2 [98] and GK [79], as well as leptin and insulin receptors [28, 83, 241]. These characteristics make NPY and POMC neurons able to sense not only glucose, but many other metabolic signals from the periphery that arrive to the CNS [56]. In addition to the hormones and metabolites mentioned above, some of the GE neurons of the

Arc and VMH neurons also respond to neurotransmitters and peptides, including monoamines [242], GABA [29], vasopressin, and oxytocin [243]. GI neurons have been show to possess similar metabolic integrator capacities: GI neurons of the LH respond to signals transmitted from the liver, as well as to taste, odour and the rewarding properties of the food [32, 37]. GI neuronal firing rate is also modulated by catecholamines [37], serotonin [244], opioids [245] and glutamate[32]. Additionally, GI neurons situated in the NTS are able to integrate internal metabolic and neural signals, and their firing rate is altered by afferent vagal signals from the liver [48] and by catecholamines released by local neurons [54].

Chapter X

Conclusion

The brain has evolved a mechanism able to sense the changes in ambient glucose levels, most probably due to its rely on glucose as a primary energetic substrate. At molecular level, the mechanism of GE neurons is similar to that described in pancreatic β-cells, consisting in GLUT2, GK, and the K_{ATP} channel. However, in GI neurons, other actors seems to be involved in the detection of glucose, such as AMPK, Na^+-K^+-ATPase, chloride channels, and tandem pore K^+ channels. The involvement of glucosensing neurons in glucose homeostasis and counterregulatory response to hypoglycemia, as well as its impairment in the T1DM condition, is today well accepted. However, whether changes in glucose circulating may elicit feeding responses through glucosensing neurons with physiological relevance or not remain to be elucidated. In this sense, glucosensing neurons have been described not only as able to detect changes in glucose levels, but also in many other metabolites and hormones that influence its final response. These characteristics make glucosensing neurons an attractive model of neurons able to receive inputs from the periphery and other central regions, integrate that information and generate a final response in order to maintain glucose homeostasis between the narrow physiological ranges.

References

[1] Lam CK, Chari M, Lam TK. CNS regulation of glucose homeostasis. *Physiology* (Bethesda). 2009 Jun;24:159-70.

[2] Pocai A, Lam TKT, Obici S, Gutiérrez-Ju rez R, Muse ED, Arduini A, et al. Restoration of hypothalamic lipid sensing normalizes energy and glucose homeostasis in overfed rats. *J. Clin. Invest.* 2006;116:1081-91.

[3] Ono H, Pocai A, Wang Y, Sakoda H, Asano T, Backer JM, et al. Activation of hypothalamic S6 kinase mediates diet-induced hepatic insulin resistance in rats. *J. Clin. Invest.* 2008 Aug;118(8):2959-68.

[4] Morrison CD, Morton GJ, Niswender KD, Gelling RW, Schwartz MW. Leptin inhibits hypothalamic Npy and Agrp gene expression via a mechanism that requires phosphatidylinositol 3-OH-kinase signaling. *Am. J. Physiol. Endocrinol. Metab.* 2005 Dec;289(6):E1051-7.

[5] Coppari R, Ichinose M, Lee CE, Pullen AE, Kenny CD, McGovern RA, et al. The hypothalamic arcuate nucleus: a key site for mediating leptin's effects on glucose homeostasis and locomotor activity. *Cell* Metab. 2005 Jan;1(1):63-72.

[6] Wild S, Roglic G, Green A, Sicree R, King H. Global prevalence of diabetes: estimates for the year 2000 and projections for 2030. *Diabetes Care.* 2004 May;27(5):1047-53.

[7] Marty N, Dallaporta M, Thorens B. Brain glucose sensing, counterregulation, and energy homeostasis. *Physiology.* 2007;22:241-51.

[8] Lee DH, Chung MY, Lee JU, Kang DG, Paek YW. Changes of glucose transporters in the cerebral adaptation to hypoglycemia. *Diabetes Res. Clin. Pract.* 2000 Jan;47(1):15-23.

[9]   Boyle PJ. Alterations in brain glucose uptake and hypoglycaemia unawareness. *Diabetes Nutr. Metab.* 2002 Oct;15(5):334-40; discussion 40, 62.

[10]   Loose NL, Rudloff E, Kirby R. Hypoglycemia and its effect on the brain. *J.Vet. Emerg. Crit. Care.* 2008;18(3):223-34.

[11]   Dwyer D. Glucose metabolism in the brain. Bradley MJ, Harris, R.A., Jenner, P. , editor: Accademic Press; 2002.

[12]   Pellerin L, Pellegri G, Bittar PG, Charnay Y, Bouras C, Martin JL, et al. Evidence supporting the existence of an activity-dependent astrocyte-neuron lactate shuttle. *Dev. Neurosci.* 1998;20(4-5):291-9.

[13]   Dringen R. Metabolism and functions of glutathione in brain. *Prog. Neurobiol.* 2000 Dec;62(6):649-71.

[14]   Bartnik BL, Sutton RL, Fukushima M, Harris NG, Hovda DA, Lee SM. Upregulation of pentose phosphate pathway and preservation of tricarboxylic acid cycle flux after experimental brain injury. *J. Neurotrauma.* 2005 Oct;22(10):1052-65.

[15]   Dienel GA. Energy metabolism in the central nervous system. In: Edvinsson L, Krause DN, editors. Cerebral Blood Flow and Metabolism. 2nd ed. Philadelphia: Lippincott Williams and Wilkins; 2001. p. 140-61.

[16]   Seaquist ER, Gruetter R. Brain glycogen: an insulin-sensitive carbohydrate store. *Diabetes. Nutr. Metab.* 2002 Oct;15(5):285-9; discussion 9-90.

[17]   Brown AM, Sickmann HM, Fosgerau K, Lund TM, Schousboe A, Waagepetersen HS, et al. Astrocyte glycogen metabolism is required for neural activity during aglycemia or intense stimulation in mouse white matter. *J. Neurosci. Res.* 2005 Jan 1-15;79(1-2):74-80.

[18]   Gruetter R. Glycogen: the forgotten cerebral energy store. *J. Neurosci. Res.* 2003 Oct 15;74(2):179-83.

[19]   Bernard C. Chiens rendu diabetiques. *C R Soc. Biol.* 1849;1:60-4.

[20]   Mayer J. Glucostatic mechanism of regulation of food intake. *N. Engl. J. Med.* 1953 Jul 2;249(1):13-6.

[21]   Stellar E. The physiology of motivation. *Psychol. Rev.* 1954 Jan;61(1):5-22.

[22]   Oomura Y, Kimura K, Ooyama H, Maeo T, Iki M, Kuniyoshi M. Reciprocal activities of the ventromedial and lateral hypothalamic areas of cats. *Science.* 1964;143:484-5.

[23]   Anand BK, Chhina GS, Sharme KN, Dua S, Singh B. Activity of single neurons in the hypothalamus feeding centers: effect of glucose. *Am. J. Physiol.* 1964;207:1146-54.

[24] Song Z, Levin BE, McArdle JJ, Bakhos N, Routh VH. Convergence of pre- and postsynaptic influences on glucosensing neurons in the ventromedial hypothalamic nucleus. *Diabetes* 2001;50(12):2673-81.

[25] Silver IA, Erecinska M. Glucose-induced intracellular ion changes in sugar-sensitive hypothalamic neurons. *J. Neurophysiol.* 1998;79(4):1733-45.

[26] Funahashi H, Yada T, Muroya S, Takigawa M, Ryushi T, Horie S, et al. The effect of leptin on feeding-regulating neurons in the rat hypothalamus. *Neurosci. Lett.* 1999;264(1-3):117-20.

[27] Muroya S, Yada T, Shioda S, Takigawa M. Glucose-sensitive neurons in the rat arcuate nucleus contain neuropeptide Y. *Neurosci. Lett.* 1999;264(1-3):113-6.

[28] Cowley MA, Smart JL, Rubinstein M, Cerdan MG, Diano S, Horvath TL, et al. Leptin activates anorexigenic POMC neurons through a neural network in the arcuate nucleus. *Nature.* 2001;411(6836):480-4.

[29] Kow LM, Pfaff DW. Responses of hypothalamic paraventricular neurons *in vitro* to norepinephrine and other feeding-relevant agents. *Physiol. Behav.* 1989;46(2):265-71.

[30] Nagai K, Niijima A, Nagai N, Hibino H, Chun SJ, Shimizu K, et al. Bilateral lesions of the hypothalamic suprachiasmatic nucleus eliminated sympathetic response to intracranial injection of 2-deoxy-D-glucose and VIP rescued this response. *Brain Res. Bull.* 1996;39(5):293-7.

[31] Hall AC, Hoffmaster RM, Stern EL, Harrington ME, Bickar D. Suprachiasmatic nucleus neurons are glucose sensitive. *J. Biol. Rhythms.* 1997 Oct;12(5):388-400.

[32] Aou S, Takaki A, Karadi Z, Hori T, Nishino H, Oomura Y. Functional heterogeneity of the monkey lateral hypothalamus in the control of feeding. *Brain Res. Bull.* 1991 Sep-Oct;27(3-4):451-5.

[33] Oomura Y, Nakamura T, Sugimori M, Yamada Y. Effect of free fatty acid on the rat lateral hypothalamic neurons. *Physiol. Behav.* 1975;14(04):483-6.

[34] Griffond B, Risold PY, Jacquemard C, Colard C, Fellmann D. Insulin-induced hypoglycemia increases preprohypocretin (orexin) mRNA in the rat lateral hypothalamic area. *Neurosci. Lett.* 1999 Mar 5;262(2):77-80.

[35] Orsini JC, Himmi T, Wiser AK, Perrin J. Local versus indirect action of glucose on the lateral hypothalamic neurons sensitive to glycemic level. *Brain Res. Bull.* 1990 Jul;25(1):49-53.

[36] Adachi A, Shimizu N, Oomura Y, Kobashi M. Convergence of hepatoportal glucose-sensitive afferent signals to glucose-sensitive units within the nucleus of the solitary tract. *Neurosci. Lett.* 1984;46(2):215-8.

[37] Karadi Z, Oomura Y, Nishino H, Scott TR, Lenard L, Aou S. Responses of lateral hypothalamic glucose-sensitive and glucose-insensitive neurons to chemical stimuli in behaving rhesus monkeys. *J. Neurophysiol.* 1992 Feb;67(2):389-400.

[38] Shoji S. Glucose regulation of synaptic transmission in the dorsolateral septal nucleus of the rat. *Synapse.* 1992 Dec;12(4):322-32.

[39] Nakano Y, Oomura Y, Lenard L, Nishino H, Aou S, Yamamoto T, et al. Feeding-related activity of glucose- and morphine-sensitive neurons in the monkey amygdala. *Brain. Res.* 1986;399(1):167-72.

[40] Lee K, Dixon AK, Freeman TC, Richardson PJ. Identification of an ATP-sensitive potassium channel current in rat striatal cholinergic interneurones. *J. Physiol.* 1998 Jul 15;510 (Pt 2):441-53.

[41] Lee K, Dixon AK, Rowe IC, Ashford ML, Richardson PJ. The high-affinity sulphonylurea receptor regulates KATP channels in nerve terminals of the rat motor cortex. *J. Neurochem.* 1996 Jun;66(6):2562-71.

[42] Liss B, Bruns R, Roeper J. Alternative sulfonylurea receptor expression defines metabolic sensitivity of K-ATP channels in dopaminergic midbrain neurons. *EMBO J.* 1999;18(4):833-46.

[43] During MJ, Leone P, Davis KE, Kerr D, Sherwin RS. Glucose modulates rat substantia nigra GABA release in vivo via ATP-sensitive potassium channels. *J. Clin. Invest.* 1995 May;95(5):2403-8.

[44] Roper J, Ashcroft FM. Metabolic inhibition and low internal ATP activate K-ATP channels in rat dopaminergic substantia nigra neurones. *Pflugers Arch.* 1995 May;430(1):44-54.

[45] Levin BE. Glucose-regulated dopamine release from substantia nigra neurons. *Brain Res.* 2000 Aug 25;874(2):158-64.

[46] Finta EP, Harms L, Sevcik J, Fischer HD, Illes P. Effects of potassium channel openers and their antagonists on rat locus coeruleus neurones. *Br. J. Pharmacol.* 1993 Jun;109(2):308-15.

[47] Dallaporta M, Perrin J, Orsini JC. Involvement of adenosine triphosphate-sensitive K^+ channels in glucose-sensing in the rat solitary tract nucleus. *Neurosci. Lett.* 2000;278(1-2):77-80.

[48] Mizuno Y, Oomura Y. Glucose responding neurons in the nucleus tractus solitarius of the rat: *in vitro* study. *Brain Res.* 1984;307(1-2):109-16.

[49] Karschin A, Brockhaus J, Ballanyi K. K_{ATP} channel formation by the sulphonylurea receptors SUR1 with Kir6.2 subunits in rat dorsal vagal neurons *in situ. J. Physiol.* 1998 Jun 1;509 (Pt 2)·339-46.

[50] Adachi A, Kobashi M, Miyoshi N, Tsukamoto G. Chemosensitive neurons in the area postrema of the rat and their possible functions. *Brain Res Bull.* 1991 Jan;26(1):137-40.

[51] Levin BE, Dunn-Meynell AA, Routh VH. CNS sensing and regulation of peripheral glucose levels. *Int. Rev. Neurobiol.* 2002;51:219-58.

[52] Ritter S, Dinh TT. 2-Mercaptoacetate and 2-deoxy-D-glucose induce Fos-like immunoreactivity in rat brain. *Brain Res.* 1994 Mar 28;641(1):111-20.

[53] Briski KP, Sylvester PW. Co-distribution of Fos- and mu opioid receptor immunoreactivity within the rat septopreoptic area and hypothalamus during acute glucose deprivation: effects of the mu receptor antagonist CTOP. *Neurosci. Lett.* 2001 Jun 29;306(3):141-4.

[54] Dallaporta M, Himmi T, Perrin J, Orsini JC. Solitary tract nucleus sensitivity to moderate changes in glucose level. *Neuroreport.* 1999;10(12):2657-60.

[55] Yang XJ, Kow LM, Pfaff DW, Mobbs CV. Metabolic pathways that mediate inhibition of hypothalamic neurons by glucose. *Diabetes.* 2004;53 67-73.

[56] Levin BE, Routh VH, Kang L, Sanders NM, Dunn-Meynell AA. Neuronal glucosensing. What do we know after 50 years? *Diabetes.* 2004;53 2521-8.

[57] Thorens B, Sarkar HK, Kaback HR, Lodish HF. Cloning and functional expression in bacteria of a novel glucose transporter present in liver, intestine, kidney, and beta-pancreatic islet cells. *Cell.* 1988;55(2):281-90.

[58] Schuit F, Moens K, Heimberg H, Pipeleers D. Cellular origin of hexokinase in pancreatic islets. *J. Biol. Chem.* 1999;274:32803-9.

[59] Detimary P, Dejonghe S, Ling Z, Pipeleers D, Schuit F, Henquin JC. The changes in adenine nucleotides measured in glucose-stimulated rodent islets occur in beta cells but not in alpha cells and are also observed in human islets. *J. Biol. Chem.* 1998;273(51):33905-8.

[60] Schuit FC, Huypens P, Heimberg H, Pipeleers DG. Glucose sensing in pancreatic β-cells. A model for the study of other glucose-regulated cells in gut, pancreas, and hypothalamus. *Diabetes.* 2001;50:1-11.

[61] Heimberg H, De Vos A, Vandercammen A, van Schaftingen E, Pipeleers D, Schuit F. Heterogeneity in glucose sensitivity among pancreatic beta-

cells is correlated to differences in glucose phosphorylation rather than glucose transport. *EMBO J.*. 1993;12(7):2873-9.

[62] Velho G, Froguel P, Clement K, Pueyo ME, Rakotoambinina B, Zouali H, et al. Primary pancreatic beta-cell secretory defect caused by mutations in glucokinase gene in kindreds of maturity onset diabetes of the young. *Lancet.* 1992;340(8817):444-8.

[63] Postic C, Shiota M, Niswender KD, Jetton TL, Chen Y, Moates JM, et al. Dual roles for glucokinase in glucose homeostasis as determined by liver and pancreatic beta cell-specific gene knock-outs using Cre recombinase. *J. Biol. Chem.* 1999;274(1):305-15.

[64] Prentki M. New insights into pancreatic beta-cell metabolic signaling in insulin secretion. *Eur. J. Endocrinol.* 1996 Mar;134(3):272-86.

[65] Aguilar-Bryan L, Bryan J. Molecular biology of adenosine triphosphate-sensitive potassium channels. *Endocr. Rev.* 1999;20(2):101-35.

[66] Tucker SJ, Gribble FM, Proks P, Trapp S, Ryder TJ, Haug T, et al. Molecular determinants of K_{ATP} channel inhibition by ATP. *EMBO J.* 1998;17(12):3290-6.

[67] Nichols CG, Shyng SL, Nestorowicz A, Glaser B, Clement JP, González G, et al. Adenosine diphosphate as an intracellular regulator of insulin secretion. *Science.* 1996;272(5269):1785-7.

[68] Ashcroft FM, Proks P, Smith PA, Ammala C, Bokvist K, Rorsman P. Stimulus-secretion coupling in pancreatic beta cells. *J. Cell Biochem.* 1994;55 Suppl:54-65.

[69] Yang XJ, Kow LM, Funabashi T, Mobbs CV. Hypothalamic glucose sensor, similarities to and differences from pancreatic β-cell mechanisms. *Diabetes.* 1999;48:1763-72.

[70] Kang L, Routh VH, Kuzhikandathil EV, Gaspers LD, Levin BE. Physiological and molecular characteristics of rat hypothalamic ventromedial nucleus glucosensing neurons. *Diabetes.* 2004;53:549-59.

[71] Vannucci SJ, Maher F, Simpson IA. Glucose transporter proteins in brain: delivery of glucose to neurons and glia. *Glia.* 1997;21(1):2-21.

[72] González JA, Reimann F, Burdakov D. Dissociation between sensing and metabolism of glucose in sugar sensing neurones. *J. Physiol.* 2009 Jan 15;587(Pt 1):41-8.

[73] O'Malley D, Reimann F, Simpson AK, Gribble FM. Sodium-coupled glucose cotransporters contribute to hypothalamic glucose sensing. *Diabetes.* 2006 Dec;55(12):3381-6.

[74] Díez-Sampedro A, Hirayama BA, Osswald C, Gorboulev V, Baumgarten K, Volk C, et al. A glucose sensor hiding in a family of transporters. *Proc. Natl. Acad. Sci. USA.* 2003;100:11753-8.

[75] Dunn-Meynell AA, Routh VH, Kang L, Gaspers L, Levin BE. Glucokinase is the likely mediator of glucosensing in both glucose-excited and glucose-inhibited central neurons. *Diabetes.* 2002;51:2056-65.

[76] Roncero I, Álvarez E, Vázquez P, Blázquez E. Functional glucokinase isoforms are expressed in rat brain. *J. Neurochem.* 2000;74(5):1848-57.

[77] Levin BE, Routh, V., Sanders, L.K., Dunn-Meynell, A. Anatomy, physiology and regulation of glucokinase as a brain glucosensor. In: Matschinsky FM, Magnuson MA, editors. Glucokinase and glycemic disease: from basics to novel therapeutics. Basel: Karger; 2004. p. 301-12.

[78] Matschinsky FM. Banting Lecture 1995. A lesson in metabolic regulation inspired by the glucokinase glucose sensor paradigm. *Diabetes.* 1996 Feb;45(2):223-41.

[79] Lynch RM, Tompkins LS, Brooks HL, Dunn-Meynell AA, Levin BE. Localization of glucokinase gene expression in the rat brain. *Diabetes.* 2000;49:693-700.

[80] Sanz C, Roncero I, Vázquez P, Navas MA, Blázquez E. Effects of glucose and insulin on glucokinase activity in rat hypothalamus. *J. Endocrinol.* 2007;193:259-67.

[81] Parmentier-Batteur S, Jin K, Xie L, Mao XO, Greenberg DA. DNA microarray analysis of cannabinoid signaling in mouse brain *in vivo.* *Mol. Pharmacol.* 2002 Oct;62(4):828-35.

[82] Dunn-Meynell AA, Govek E, Levin BE. Intracarotid glucose selectively increases Fos-like immunoreactivity in paraventricular, ventromedial and dorsomedial nuclei neurons. *Brain Res.* 1997;748(1-2):100-6.

[83] Wang R, Liu X, Hentges ST, Dunn-Meynell AA, Levin BE, Wang W, et al. The regulation of glucose-excited neurons in the hypothalamic arcuate nucleus by glucose and feeding-relevant peptides. *Diabetes.* 2004;53:1959-65.

[84] Kang L, Dunn-Meynell AA, Routh VH, Liu X, Levin BE. Knockdown of GK mRNA with GK RNA interference (RNAi) blocks ventromedial hypothalamic (VMH) neuronal glucosensing. *Diabetes.* 2004;53(Suppl. 2):A43.

[85] Iynedjian PB. Molecular physiology of mammalian glucokinase. *Cell. Mol. Life Sci.* 2008 Aug 26.

[86]   Vandercammen A, van Schaftingen E. Competitive inhibition of liver
       glucokinase by its regulatory protein. *Eur. J. Biochem.* 1991;200(2):545-
       51.

[87]   Álvarez E, Roncero I, Chowen JA, Vázquez P, Blázquez E. Evidence
       that glucokinase regulatory protein is expressed and interacts with
       glucokinase in rat brain. *J. Neurochem.* 2002 Jan;80(1):45-53.

[88]   Massa L, Baltrusch S, Okar DA, Lange AJ, Lenzen S, Tiedge M.
       Interaction of 6-phosphofructo-2-kinase/fructose-2,6-bisphosphatase
       (PFK-2/FBPase-2) with glucokinase activates glucose phosphorylation
       and glucose metabolism in insulin-producing cells. *Diabetes.* 2004
       Apr;53(4):1020-9.

[89]   Miki T, Nagashima K, Tashiro F, Kotake K, Yoshitomi H, Tamamoto A,
       et al. Defective insulin secretion and enhanced insulin action in K_{ATP}
       channel-deficient mice. *Proc. Natl. Acad. Sci. U.S.A.* 1998 Sep
       1;95(18):10402-6.

[90]   Miki T, Liss B, Minami K, Shiuchi T, Saraya A, Kashima Y, et al. ATP-
       sensitive K^+ channels in the hypothalamus are essential for the
       maintenance of glucose homeostasis. *Nat, Neurosci.* 2001;4:507-12.

[91]   Ohno-Shosaku T, Yamamoto C. Identification of an ATP-sensitive K^+
       channel in rat cultured cortical neurons. *Pflugers Arch.* 1992
       Dec;422(3):260-6.

[92]   Zawar C, Plant TD, Schirra C, Konnerth A, Neumcke B. Cell-type
       specific expression of ATP-sensitive potassium channels in the rat
       hippocampus. *J. Physiol.* 1999 Jan 15;514 (Pt 2):327-41.

[93]   Ashford ML, Boden PR, Treherne JM. Tolbutamide excites rat
       glucoreceptive ventromedial hypothalamic neurones by indirect
       inhibition of ATP-K^+ channels. *Br. J. Pharmacol.* 1990;101(3):531-40.

[94]   Levin BE, Dunn-Meynell AA, Routh VH. Brain glucose sensing and
       body energy homeostasis: role in obesity and diabetes. *Am. J. Physiol.
       Regul. Integr. Comp. Physiol.* 1999;276:R1223-R31.

[95]   Aguilar-Bryan L, Clement JP, González G, Kunjilwar K, Babenko A,
       Bryan J. Toward understanding the assembly and structure of K_{ATP}
       channels. *Physiol. Rev.* 1998;78(1):227-45.

[96]   Inagaki N, Gonoi T, Clement JP, Namba N, Inazawa J, González G, et
       al. Reconstitution of IKATP: an inward rectifier subunit plus the
       sulfonylurea receptor. *Science.* 1995;270(5239):1166-70.

[97]   Peyrollier K, Heron L, Virsolvy-Vergine A, Le Cam A, Bataille D.
       Alpha endosulfine is a novel molecule, structurally related to a family of

phosphoproteins. Biochem *Biophys. Res. Commun.* 1996 Jun 25,223(3):583-6,

[98] Dunn-Meynell AA, Rawson NE, Levin DE. Distribution and phenotype of neurons containing the ATP-sensitive K$^+$ channel in rat brain. *Brain Res.* 1998;814(1-2):41-54.

[99] Levin BE, Brown KL, Dunn-Meynell AA. Differential effects of diet and obesity on high and low affinity sulfonylurea binding sites in the rat brain. *Brain Res.* 1996;739(1-2):293-300.

[100] Dunn-Meynell AA, Routh VH, McArdle JJ, Levin BE. Low-affinity sulfonylurea binding sites reside on neuronal cell bodies in the brain. *Brain Res.* 1997;745(1-2):1-9.

[101] Sellers AJ, Boden PR, Ashford ML. Lack of effect of potassium channel openers on ATP-modulated potassium channels recorded from rat ventromedial hypothalamic neurones. *Br. J. Pharmacol.* 1992 Dec;107(4):1068-74.

[102] Routh VH, McArdle JJ, Levin BE. Phosphorylation modulates the activity of the ATP-sensitive K$^+$ channel in the ventromedial hypothalamic nucleus. *Brain Res.* 1997;778(1):107-19.

[103] Lee K, Dixon AK, Rowe IC, Ashford ML, Richardson PJ. Direct demonstration of sulphonylurea-sensitive K$_{ATP}$ channels on nerve terminals of the rat motor cortex. *Br. J. Pharmacol.* 1995 Jun;115(3):385-7.

[104] Lee K, Brownhill V, Richardson PJ. Antidiabetic sulphonylureas stimulate acetylcholine release from striatal cholinergic interneurones through inhibition of K(ATP) channel activity. *J. Neurochem.* 1997 Oct;69(4):1774-6.

[105] Song Z, Routh VH. Differential effects of glucose and lactate on glucosensing neurons in the ventromedial hypothalamic nucleus. *Diabetes.* 2005;54:15-22.

[106] Fioramonti X, Lorsignol A, Taupignon A, Pénicaud L. A new ATP-sensitive K$^+$ channel-independent mechanism is involved in glucose-excited neurons of mouse arcuate nucleus. *Diabetes.* 2004;53(11):2767-75.

[107] Oomura Y, Ooyama H, Sugimori M, Nakamura T, Yamada Y. Glucose inhibition of the glucose-sensitive neurone in the rat lateral hypothalamus. *Nature.* 1974;247(439):284-6.

[108] Routh VH. Glucose-sensing neurons: are they physiologically relevant? *Physiol. Behav.* 2002;76(3):403-13.

[109] Burdakov D, González JA. Physiological functions of glucose-inhibited neurons. *Acta Physiol.* (Oxf). 2009 Oct 28;195:71-8.

[110] Fioramonti X, Contie S, Song Z, Routh VH, Lorsignol A, Pénicaud L. Characterization of glucosensing neuron subpopulations in the arcuate nucleus: integration in neuropeptide Y and pro-opio melanocortin networks? *Diabetes.* 2007 May;56(5):1219-27.

[111] Burdakov D, Jensen LT, Alexopoulos H, Williams RH, Fearon IM, O'Kelly I, et al. Tandem-pore K^+ channels mediate inhibition of orexin neurons by glucose. *Neuron.* 2006 Jun 1;50(5):711-22.

[112] Pellerin L, Magistretti PJ. Glutamate uptake into astrocytes stimulates aerobic glycolysis: a mechanism coupling neuronal activity to glucose utilization. *Proc. Natl. Acad. Sci. U.S.A.* 1994;91:10625-9.

[113] Wender R, Brown AM, Fern R, Swanson RA, Farrell K, Ransom BR. Astrocytic glycogen influences axon function and survival during glucose deprivattion in central white matter. *J. Neurosci.* 2000;200:6804-10.

[114] Pierre K, Pellerin L, Debernardi R, Riederer BM, Magistretti PJ. Cell-specific localization of monocarboxylate transporters, MCT1 and MCT2, in thea dult mouse brain revealed by double immunohistochemical labeling and confocal microscopy. *Neuroscience.* 2000;100:617-27.

[115] Ainscow EK, Mirshamsi S, Tang T, Ashford MLJ, Rutter GA. Dynamic imaging of free cytosolic ATP concentration duyring fuel sensing by rat hypothalamic neurons: evidence for ATP-independent control of ATP-sensitive K^+ channels. *J. Physiol.* 2002;544:429-45.

[116] Pellerin L, Magistretti PJ. Neuroenergetics: calling upon astrocytes to satisfy hungry neurons. *Neuroscientist.* 2004;10(1):53-62.

[117] Lam TKT, Gutiérrez-Juárez R, Pocai A, Rossetti L. Regulation of blood glucose by hypothalamic pyruvate metabolism. *Science.* 2005;309:943-7.

[118] Guillod-Maximin E, Lorsignol A, Alquier T, Penicaud L. Acute intracarotid glucose injection towards the brain induces specific c-fos activation in hypothalamic nuclei: involvement of astrocytes in cerebral glucose-sensing in rats. *J. Neuroendocrinol.* 2004 May;16(5):464-71.

[119] Briski KP, Patil GD. Induction of Fos immunoreactivity labeling in rat forebrain metabolic loci by caudal fourth ventricular infusion of the monocarboxylate transporter inhibitor, alpha-cyano-4-hydroxycinnamic acid. *Neuroendocrinology.* 2005;82(1):49-57.

[120] Patil GD, Briski KP. Lactate is a critical "sensed" variable in caudal hindbrain monitoring of CNS metabolic stasis. *Am. J. Physiol. Regul. Integr. Comp. Physiol.* 2005;289:R1777-R86.

[121] Patil GD, Briski KP. Transcriptional activation of nucleus tractus solitarii/area postrema catecholaminergic neurons by pharmacological inhibition of caudal hindbrain monocarboxylate transporter function. *Neuroendocrinology.* 2005;81(2):96-102.

[122] Vavaiya KV, Briski KP. Caudal hindbrain lactate infusion alters glucokinase, SUR1, and neuronal substrate fuel transporter gene expression in the dorsal vagal complex, lateral hypothalamic area, and ventromedial nucleus hypothalamus of hypoglycemic male rats. *Brain Res.* 2007;1176:62-70.

[123] Bouzier-Sore AK, Voisin P, Canioni P, Magistretti PJ, Pellerin L. Lactate is a preferential oxidative energy substrate over glucose for neurons in culture. *J. Cereb. Blood Flow Metab.* 2003;23(11):1298-306.

[124] Cone RD, Cowley MA, Butler AA, Fan W, Marks DL, Low MJ. The arcuate nucleus as a conduit for diverse signals relevant to energy homeostasis. *Int. J. Obes. Relat. Metab. Disord.* 2001;25 Suppl 5:S63-S7.

[125] Ibrahim N, Bosch MA, Smart JL, Qiu J, Rubinstein M, Ronnekleiv OK, et al. Hypothalamic proopiomelanocortin neurons are glucose responsive and express K(ATP) channels. *Endocrinology.* 2003;144(4):1331-40.

[126] Cai XJ, Evans ML, Lister CA, Leslie RA, Arch JR, Wilson S, et al. Hypoglycemia activates orexin neurons and selectively increases hypothalamic orexin-B levels: responses inhibited by feeding and possibly mediated by the nucleus of the solitary tract. *Diabetes.* 2001;50(1):105-12.

[127] Moriguchi T, Sakurai T, Nambu T, Yanagisawa M, Goto K. Neurons containing orexin in the lateral hypothalamic area of the adult rat brain are activated by insulin-induced acute hypoglycemia. *Neurosci. Lett.* 1999;264:101-4.

[128] Liu XH, Morris R, Spiller D, White M, Williams G. Orexin a preferentially excites glucose-sensitive neurons in the lateral hypothalamus of the rat *in vitro*. *Diabetes.* 2001 Nov;50(11):2431-7.

[129] Muroya S, Uramura K, Sakurai T, Takigawa M, Yada T. Lowering glucose concentrations increases cytosolic Ca2+ in orexin neurons of the rat lateral hypothalamus. *Neurosci. Lett.* 2001 Aug 31;309(3):165-8.

[130] Yamanaka A, Beuckmann CT, Willie JT, Hara J, Tsujino N, Mieda M, et al. Hypothalamic orexin neurons regulate arousal according to energy balance in mice. *Neuron.* 2003;38(5):701-13.

[131] Burdakov D, Gerasimenko O, Verkhratsky A. Physiological changes in glucose differentially modulate the excitability of hypothalamic melanin-concentrating hormone and orexin neurons *in situ. J. Neurosci.* 2005 Mar 2;25(9):2429-33.

[132] Burdakov D, Luckman SM, Verkhratsky A. Glucose-sensing neurons of the hypothalamus. *Phil. Trans. R. Soc. Lond B-Biol. Sci.* 2005;360:2227-35.

[133] Sakurai T, Amemiya A, Ishii M, Matsuzaki I, Chemelli RM, Tanaka H, et al. Orexins and orexin receptors: a family of hypothalamic neuropeptides and G protein-coupled receptors that regulate feeding behavior. *Cell.* 1998 Mar 6;92(5):573-85.

[134] van den Top M, Lee K, Whyment AD, Blanks AM, Spanswick D. Orexigen-sensitive NPY/AgRP pacemaker neurons in the hypothalamic arcuate nucleus. *Nat. Neurosci.* 2004 May;7(5):493-4.

[135] Ma X, Zubcevic L, Bruning JC, Ashcroft FM, Burdakov D. Electrical inhibition of identified anorexigenic POMC neurons by orexin/hypocretin. *J. Neurosci.* 2007 Feb 14;27(7):1529-33.

[136] Muroya S, Funahashi H, Yamanaka A, Kohno D, Uramura K, Nambu T, et al. Orexins (hypocretins) directly interact with neuropeptide Y, POMC and glucose-responsive neurons to regulate Ca^{2+} signaling in a reciprocal manner to leptin: orexigenic neuronal pathways in the mediobasal hypothalamus. *Eur. J. Neurosci.* 2004 Mar;19(6):1524-34.

[137] Hara J, Beuckmann CT, Nambu T, Willie JT, Chemelli RM, Sinton CM, et al. Genetic ablation of orexin neurons in mice results in narcolepsy, hypophagia, and obesity. *Neuron.* 2001 May;30(2):345-54.

[138] Shimada M, Tritos NA, Lowell BB, Flier JS, Maratos-Flier E. Mice lacking melanin-concentrating hormone are hypophagic and lean. *Nature.* 1998 Dec 17;396(6712):670-4.

[139] Cryer PE, Fisher JN, Shamoon H. Hypoglycemia. *Diabetes Care.* 1994 Jul;17(7):734-55.

[140] Silver IA, Erecinska M. Extracellular glucose concentration in mammalian brain: continuous monitoring of changes during increased neuronal activity and upon limitation in oxygen suplly in normo-, hypo-, and hyperglycemic animals. *J. Neurosci.* 1994;14:5068-76.

[141] Paschen W, Siesjo BK, Ingvar M, Hossmann KA. Regional differences in brain glucose content in graded hypoglycemia. *Neurochem. Pathol.* 1986 Oct;5(2):131-42.

[142] McNay EC, Gold PE. Extracellular glucose concentrations in the rat hippocampus measured by zero-net-flux: effects of microdialysis flow rate, strain, and age. *J. Neurochem.* 1999 Feb;72(2):785-90.

[143] McNay EC, Gold PE. Age-related differences in hippocampal extracellular fluid glucose concentration during behavioral testing and following systemic glucose administration. *J. Gerontol. A Biol. Sci. Med. Sci.* 2001 Feb;56(2):B66-71.

[144] McNay EC, McCarty RC, Gold PE. Fluctuations in brain glucose concentration during behavioral testing: dissociations between brain areas and between brain and blood. *Neurobiol. Lear Mem.* 2001;75(3):325-37.

[145] McCrimmon RJ, Fan X, Ding Y, Zhu W, Jacob RJ, Sherwin RS. Potential role for AMP-activated protein kinase in hypoglycemia sensing in the ventromedial hypothalamus. *Diabetes.* 2004 Aug;53(8):1953-8.

[146] Taborsky Jr GJ, Ahren B, Havel PJ. Autonomic mediation of glucagon secretion during hypoglycemia: implications for impaired alpha-cell responses in type 1 diabetes. *Diabetes.* 1998 Jul;47(7):995-1005.

[147] Cryer PE. Diverse causes of hypoglycemia-associated autonomic failure in diabetes. *N. Engl. J. Med.* 2004;350(22):2272-9.

[148] Mitrakou A, Ryan C, Veneman T, Mokan M, Jenssen T, Kiss I, et al. Hierarchy of glycemic thresholds for counterregulatory hormone secretion, symptoms, and cerebral dysfunction. *Am. J. Physiol. Endocrinol. Metab.* 1991;260(1 Pt 1):E67-E74.

[149] de Vries MG, Lawson MA, Beverly JL. Hypoglycemia-induced noradrenergic activation in the VMH is a result of decreased ambient glucose. *Am. J. Physiol. Regul. Integr. Comp. Physiol.* 2005;289:R977-R81.

[150] Hevener AL, Bergman RN, Donovan CM. Portal vein afferents are critical for the sympathoadrenal response to hypoglycemia. *Diabetes.* 2000;49(1):8-12.

[151] Frizzell RT, Jones EM, Davis SN, Biggers DW, Myers SR, Connolly CC, et al. Counterregulation during hypoglycemia is directed by widespread brain regions. *Diabetes.* 1993;42(9):1253-61.

[152] Kennan RP, Takahashi K, Pan C, Shamoon H, Pan JW. Human cerebral blood flow and metabolism in acute insulin-induced hypoglycemia. *J. Cereb. Blood Flow Metab.* 2005 Apr;25(4):527-34.

[153] Simpson IA, Appel NM, Hokari M, Oki J, Holman GD, Maher F, et al. Blood-brain barrier glucose transporter: effects of hypo- and hyperglycemia revisited. *J. Neurochem.* 1999 Jan;72(1):238-47.

[154] Yao H, Sadoshima S, Nishimura Y, Fujii K, Oshima M, Ishitsuka T, et al. Cerebrospinal fluid lactate in patients with diabetes mellitus and hypoglycaemic coma. *J. Neurol. Neurosurg. Psychiatry.* 1989 Mar;52(3):372-5.

[155] Beverly JL, De Vries MG, Bouman SD, Arseneau LM. Noradrenergic and GABAergic systems in the medial hypothalamus are activated during hypoglycemia. *Am. J. Physiol. Regul. Integr. Comp. Physiol.* 2001 Feb;280(2):R563-9.

[156] Biggers DW, Myers SR, Neal D, Stinson R, Cooper NB, Jaspan JB, et al. Role of brain in counterregulation of insulin-induced hypoglycemia in dogs. *Diabetes.* 1989;38(1):7-16.

[157] Borg WP, Sherwin RS, During MJ, Borg MA, Shulman GI. Local ventromedial hypothalamus glucopenia triggers counterregulatory hormone release. *Diabetes.* 1995;44(2):180-4.

[158] Borg MA, Sherwin RS, Borg WP, Tamborlane WV, Shulman GI. Local ventromedial hypothalamus glucose perfusion blocks counterregulation during systemic hypoglycemia in awake rats. *J. Clin. Invest.* 1997;99(2):361-5.

[159] Borg WP, During MJ, Sherwin RS, Borg MA, Brines ML, Shulman GI. Ventromedial hypothalamic lesions in rats suppress counterregulatory responses to hypoglycemia. *J. Clin. Invest.* 1994;93:1677-82.

[160] McCrimmon RJ, Song Z, Cheng H, McNay EC, Weikart-Yeckel C, Fan X, et al. Corticotrophin-releasing factor receptors within the ventromedial hypothalamus regulate hypoglycemia-induced hormonal counterregulation. *J. Clin. Invest.* 2006 Jun;116(6):1723-30.

[161] Cryer PE. Mechanisms of sympathoadrenal failure and hypoglycemia in diabetes. *J. Clin. Invest.* 2006 Jun;116(6):1470-3.

[162] Egawa M, Yoshimatsu H, Bray GA. Lateral hypothalamic injection of 2-deoxy-D-glucose suppresses sympathetic activity. *Am. J. Physiol. Regul. Integr. Comp. Physiol.* 1989 Dec;257(6 Pt 2):1386-92.

[163] Yoshimatsu H, Egawa M, Bray GA. Adrenal sympathetic nerve activity in response to hypothalamic injections of 2-deoxy-D-glucose. *Am. J. Physiol. Regul. Integr. Comp. Physiol.* 1991 Oct;261(4 Pt 2):875-81.

[164] Ritter S, Bugarith K, Dinh TT. Immunotoxic destruction of distinct catecholamine subgroups produces selective impairment of

glucoregulatory responses and neuronal activation. *J. Comp. Neurol.* 2001 Apr 2;432(2):197-216.

[165] Ritter RC, Slusser PG, Stone S. Glucoreceptors controlling feeding and blood glucose: location in the hindbrain. *Science.* 1981;213(4506):451-2.

[166] Fraley GS, Ritter S. Immunolesion of norepinephrine and epinephrine afferents to medial hypothalamus alters basal and 2-deoxy-D-glucose-induced neuropeptide Y and agouti gene-related protein messenger ribonucleic acid expression in the arcuate nucleus. *Endocrinology.* 2003 Jan;144(1):75-83.

[167] Ritter S, Dinh TT, Zhang Y. Localization of hindbrain glucoreceptive sites controlling food intake and blood glucose. *Brain Res.* 2000;856:37-47.

[168] DiRocco RJ, Grill HJ. The forebrain is not essential for sympathoadrenal hyperglycemic response to glucoprivation. *Science.* 1979; 204 (4397): 1112-4.

[169] Ritter S, Llewellyn-Smith I, Dinh TT. Subgroups of hindbrain catecholamine neurons are selectively activated by 2-deoxy-D-glucose induced metabolic challenge. *Brain Res.* 1998;805(1-2):41-54.

[170] Mokan M, Mitrakou A, Veneman T, Ryan C, Korytkowski M, Cryer P, et al. Hypoglycemia unawareness in IDDM. *Diabetes Care.* 1994 Dec;17(12):1397-403.

[171] Group TDR. Epidemiology of severe hypoglycemia in the diabetes control and complications trial. The DCCT Research Group. *Am. J. Med.* 1991 Apr;90(4):450-9.

[172] McCrimmon R. The mechanisms that underlie glucose sensing during hypoglycaemia in diabetes. *Diabet. Med.* 2008 May;25(5):513-22.

[173] Borg MA, Borg WP, Tamborlane WV, Brines ML, Shulman GI, Sherwin RS. Chronic hypoglycemia and diabetes impair counterregulation induced by localized 2-deoxy-glucose perfusion of the ventromedial hypothalamus in rats. *Diabetes.* 1999 Mar;48(3):584-7.

[174] Song Z, Routh VH. Recurrent hypoglycemia reduces the glucose sensitivity of glucose-inhibited neurons in the ventromedial hypothalamus nucleus. *Am. J. Physiol. Regul. Integr. Comp. Physiol.* 2006;291 R1283-R7.

[175] McCrimmon RJ, Fan X, Cheng H, McNay E, Chan O, Shaw M, et al. Activation of AMP-activated protein kinase within the ventromedial hypothalamus amplifies counterregulatory hormone responses in rats with defective counterregulation. *Diabetes.* 2006 Jun;55(6):1755-60.

[176] Thorens B, Guillam MT, Beermann F, Burcelin R, Jaquet M. Transgenic reexpression of GLUT1 or GLUT2 in pancreatic beta cells rescues GLUT2-null mice from early death and restores normal glucose-stimulated insulin secretion. *J. Biol. Chem.* 2000;275(31):23751-8.

[177] Marty N, Dallaporta M, Foretz M, Emery M, Tarussio D, Bady I, et al. Regulation of glucagon secretion by glucose transporter type 2 (GLUT2) and astrocyte-dependent glucose sensors. *J. Clin. Invest.* 2005;115(12):3545-53.

[178] Sanders NM, Dunn-Meynell AA, Levin BE. Third ventricular alloxan reversibly impairs glucose conterregulatory responses. *Diabetes.* 2004;53 1230-6.

[179] Woods SC, McKay LD. Intraventricular alloxan eliminates feeding elicited by 2-deoxyglucose. *Science.* 1978;202(4373):1209-11.

[180] Levin BE, Becker TC, Eiki JI, Zhang BB, Dunn-Meynell AA. Ventromedial hypothalamic glucokinase is an important mediator of the counterregulatory response to insulin-induced hypoglycemia. *Diabetes.* 2008.

[181] de Vries MG, Arseneau LM, Lawson ME, Beverly JL. Extracellular glucose in rat ventromedial hypothalamus during acute and recurrent hypoglycemia. *Diabetes.* 2003 Nov;52(11):2767-73.

[182] Evans ML, McCrimmon RJ, Flanagan DE, Keshavarz T, Fan X, McNay EC, et al. Hypothalamic ATP-sensitive K^+ channels play a key role in sensing hypoglycemia and triggering counterregulatory epinephrine and glucagon responses. *Diabetes.* 2004;53(10):2542-51.

[183] McCrimmon RJ, Evans ML, Fan X, McNay EC, Chan O, Ding Y, et al. Activation of ATP-sensitive K^+ channels in the ventromedial hypothalamus amplifies counterregulatory hormone responses to hypoglycemia in normal and recurrently hypoglycemic rats. *Diabetes.* 2005;54:3169-74.

[184] Hardie DG, Carling D. The AMP-activated protein kinase: fuel gauge of the mammalian cell? *Eur. J. Biochem.* 1997 Jun 1;246(2):259-73.

[185] Han SM, Namkoong C, Jang PG, Park IS, Hong SW, Katakami H, et al. Hypothalamic AMP-activated protein kinase mediates counter-regulatory responses to hypoglycaemia in rats. *Diabetologia.* 2005;48(10):2170-8.

[186] Canabal DD, Song Z, Potian JG, Beuve A, McArdle JJ, Routh VH. Glucose, insulin, and leptin signaling pathways modulate nitric oxide synthesis in glucose-inhibited neurons in the ventromedial

hypothalamus. *Am. J. Physiol. Regul. Integr. Comp. Physiol.* 2007;292:R1418-R28.

[187] McCrimmon RJ, Shaw M, Fan X, Cheng H, Ding Y, Vella MC, et al. Key role for AMP-activated protein kinase in the ventromedial hypothalamus in regulating counterregulatory hormone responses to acute hypoglycemia. *Diabetes.* 2008 Feb;57(2):444-50.

[188] Campfield LA, Brandon P, Smith FJ. On-line continuous measurement of blood glucose and meal pattern in free-feeding rats: the role of glucose in meal initiation. *Brain Res. Bull.* 1985;14(6):605-16.

[189] Campfield LA, Smith FJ. Functional coupling between transient declines in blood glucose and feeding behavior: temporal relationships. *Brain Res. Bull.* 1986;17(3):427-33.

[190] Louis-Sylvestre J, Le Magnen J. A fall in blood glucose level precedes meal onset in free-feeding rats. *Obes. Res.* 1980;4(5):497-500.

[191] Melanson KJ, Westerterp-Plantenga MS, Campfield LA, Saris WH. Appetite and blood glucose profiles in humans after glycogen-depleting exercise. *J. Appl. Physiol.* 1999 Sep;87(3):947-54.

[192] Dunn-Meynell AA, Sanders NM, Compton D, Becker TC, Eiki J, Zhang BB, et al. Relationship among brain and blood glucose levels and spontaneous and glucoprivic feeding. *J. Neurosci.* 2009 May 27;29(21):7015-22.

[193] Ritter RC, Slusser P. 5-Thio-D-glucose causes increased feeding and hyperglycemia in the rat. *Am. J. Physiol. Endocrinol. Metab.* 1980;238:E141-E4.

[194] Novin D, VanderWeele DA, Rezek M. Infusion of 2-deoxy-D-glucose into the hepatic-portal system causes eating: evidence for peripheral glucoreceptors. *Science.* 1973 Aug 31;181(102):858-60.

[195] Miselis RR, Epstein AN. Feeding induced by intracerebroventricular 2-deoxy-D-glucose in the rat. *Am. J. Physiol.* 1975;229:1438-47.

[196] Berthoud HR, Mogenson GJ. Ingestive behavior after intracerebral and intracerebroventricular infusions of glucose and 2-deoxy-D-glucose. *Am. J. Physiol. Regul. Integr.Comp. Physiol.* 1977;233:R127-R33.

[197] Scheurink A, Ritter S. Sympathoadrenal responses to glucoprivation and lipoprivation in rats. *Physiol. Behav.* 1993 May;53(5):995-1000.

[198] Larue-Achagiotis C, Le Magnen J. Feeding rate and responses to food deprivation as a function of fasting-induced hypoglycemia. *Behav. Neurosci.* 1985 Dec;99(6):1176-80.

[199] Weigle DS, Duell PB, Connor WE, Steiner RA, Soules MR, Kuijper JL. Effect of fasting, refeeding, and dietary fat restriction on plasma leptin levels. *J. Clin. Endocrinol. Metab.* 1997 Feb;82(2):561-5.

[200] Klein S, Wolfe RR. Carbohydrate restriction regulates the adaptive response to fasting. *Am. J. Physiol. Endocrinol. Metab.* 1992 May;262(5 Pt 1):631-6.

[201] Wiater MF, Ritter S. Leptin does not attenuate the hyperphagia induced by 2-deoxy-D-glucose. *Ann. N. Y. Acad. Sci.* 1999 Nov 18;892:334-6.

[202] Bergen HT, Monkman N, Mobbs CV. Injection with gold thioglucose impairs sensitivity to glucose: evidence that glucose-responsive neurons are important for long-term regulation of body weight. *Brain Res.* 1996 Sep 23;734(1-2):332-6.

[203] Leibowitz SF, Jhanwar-Uniyal M, Dvorkin B, Makman MH. Distribution of alpha-adrenergic, beta-adrenergic and dopaminergic receptors in discrete hypothalamic areas of rat. *Brain Res.* 1982 Feb 4;233(1):97-114.

[204] Giraudo SQ, Grace MK, Billington CJ, Levine AS. Differential effects of neuropeptide Y and the mu-agonist DAMGO on 'palatability' vs. 'energy'. *Brain Res.* 1999 Jul 10;834(1-2):160-3.

[205] Kelley AE, Bless EP, Swanson CJ. Investigation of the effects of opiate antagonists infused into the nucleus accumbens on feeding and sucrose drinking in rats. *J. Pharmacol. Exp. Ther.* 1996 Sep;278(3):1499-507.

[206] Stanley BG, Magdalin W, Seirafi A, Thomas WJ, Leibowitz SF. The perifornical area: the major focus of (a) patchily distributed hypothalamic neuropeptide Y-sensitive feeding system(s). *Brain Res.* 1993 Feb 26;604(1-2):304-17.

[207] Jansen AS, Wessendorf MW, Loewy AD. Transneuronal labeling of CNS neuropeptide and monoamine neurons after pseudorabies virus injections into the stellate ganglion. *Brain Res.* 1995 Jun 12;683(1):1-24.

[208] Bady I, Marty N, Dallaporta M, Emery M, Gyger J, Tarussio D, et al. Evidence from GLUT2-null mice that glucose is a critical physiological regulator of feeding. *Diabetes.* 2006;55(4):988-95.

[209] Wan HZ, Hulsey MG, Martin RJ. Intracerebroventricular administration of antisense oligodeoxynucleotide against GLUT2 glucose transporter mRNA reduces food intake, body weight change and glucoprivic feeding response in rats. *J. Nutr.* 1998;128(2):287-91.

[210] Ritter S, Strang M. Fourth ventricular alloxan injection causes feeding but not hyperglycemia in rats. *Brain Res.* 1982;249(1):198-201.

[211] Gyte A, Pritchard LE, Jones HB, Brennand JC, White A. Reduced expression of the K_{ATP} channel subunit, Kir6.2, is associated with decreased expression of neuropeptide Y and agouti-related protein in the hypothalami of Zucker diabetic fatty rats. *J. Neuroendocrinol.* 2007 Dec;19(12):941-51.

[212] Kim MS, Lee KU. Role of hypothalamic 5'-AMP-activated protein kinase in the regulation of food intake and energy homeostasis. *J. Mol. Med.* 2005 Jul;83(7):514-20.

[213] Xue B, Kahn BB. AMPK integrates nutrient and hormonal signals to regulate food intake and energy balance through effects in the hypothalamus and peripheral tissues. *J. Physiol.* 2006;574(Pt 1):73-83.

[214] Kola B. Role of AMP-activated protein kinase in the control of appetite. *J. Neuroendocrinol.* 2008;20(7):942-51.

[215] Turnley AM, Stapleton D, Mann RJ, Witters LA, Kemp BE, Bartlett PF. Cellular distribution and developmental expression of AMP-activated protein kinase isoforms in mouse central nervous system. *J. Neurochem.* 1999;72(4):1707-16.

[216] Minokoshi Y, Alquier T, Furukawa N, Kim YB, Lee A, Xue B, et al. AMP-kinase regulates food intake by responding to hormonal and nutrient signals in the hypothalamus. *Nature.* 2004;428(6982):569-74.

[217] Andersson U, Filipsson K, Abbott CR, Woods A, Smith K, Bloom SR, et al. AMP-activated protein kinase plays a role in the control of food intake. *J. Biol. Chem.* 2004;279:12005-8.

[218] Mountjoy PD, Bailey SJ, Rutter GA. Inhibition by glucose or leptin of hypothalamic neurons expressing neuropeptide Y requires changes in AMP-activated protein kinase activity. *Diabetologia.* 2007 Jan;50(1):168-77.

[219] Korbonits M, Goldstone AP, Gueorguiev M, Grossman AB. Ghrelin: a hormone with multiple functions. *Front Neuroendocrinol.* 2004 Apr;25(1):27-68.

[220] Kola B, Hubina E, Tucci SA, Kirkham TC, Garcia EA, Mitchell SE, et al. Cannabinoids and ghrelin have both central and peripheral metabolic and cardiac effects via AMP-activated protein kinase. *J. Biol. Chem.* 2005 Jul 1;280(26):25196-201.

[221] Pagotto U, Marsicano G, Cota D, Lutz B, Pasquali R. The emerging role of the endocannabinoid system in endocrine regulation and energy balance. *Endocr. Rev.* 2006 Feb;27(1):73-100.

[222] Kubota N, Yano W, Kubota T, Yamauchi T, Itoh S, Kumagai H, et al. Adiponectin stimulates AMP-activated protein kinase in the

hypothalamus and increases food intake. *Cell Metab.* 2007 Jul;6(1):55-68.

[223] da Silva Xavier G, Leclerc I, Salt IP, Doiron B, Hardie DG, Kahn A, et al. Role of AMP-activated protein kinase in the regulation by glucose of islet beta cell gene expression. *Proc. Natl. Acad. Sci. U.S.A.* 2000 Apr 11;97(8):4023-8.

[224] da Silva Xavier G, Leclerc I, Varadi A, Tsuboi T, Moule SK, Rutter GA. Role for AMP-activated protein kinase in glucose-stimulated insulin secretion and preproinsulin gene expression. *Biochem. J.* 2003 May 1;371(Pt 3):761-74.

[225] Claret M, Smith MA, Batterham RL, Selman C, Choudhury AI, Fryer LG, et al. AMPK is essential for energy homeostasis regulation and glucose sensing by POMC and AgRP neurons. *J. Clin. Invest.* 2007;117(8):2325-36.

[226] Mountjoy PD, Rutter GA. Glucose sensing by hypothalamic neurones and pancreatic islet cells: AMPle evidence for common mechanisms? *Exp. Physiol.* 2007 Mar;92(2):311-9.

[227] Elias CF, Aschkenasi C, Lee C, Kelly J, Ahima RS, Bjorbaek C, et al. Leptin differentially regulates NPY and POMC neurons projecting to the lateral hypothalamic area. *Neuron.* 1999 Aug;23(4):775-86.

[228] Levin BE. Glucosensing neurons do more than just sense glucose. *Int. J. Obes.* 2001;25, Suppl 5 S68-S72.

[229] Minami T, Shimizu N, Duan S, Oomura Y. Hypothalamic neuronal activity responses to 3-hydroxybutyric acid, an endogenous organic acid. *Brain Res.* 1990;509(2):351-4.

[230] Migrenne S, Magnan C, Cruciani-Guglielmacci C. Fatty acid sensing and nervous control of energy homeostasis. *Diabetes Metab.* 2007 Jun;33(3):177-82.

[231] Spanswick D, Smith MA, Groppi VE, Logan SD, Ashford ML. Leptin inhibits hypothalamic neurons by activation of ATP-sensitive potassium channels. *Nature.* 1997 Dec 4;390(6659):521-5.

[232] Spanswick D, Smith MA, Mirshamsi S, Routh VH, Ashford MLJ. Insulin activates ATP-sensitive K^+ channels in hypothalamic neurons of lean, but not obese rats. *Nat. Neurosci.* 2000;3:757-8.

[233] Branstrom R, Corkey BE, Berggren PO, Larsson O. Evidence for a unique long chain acyl-CoA ester binding site on the ATP-regulated potassium channel in mouse pancreatic beta cells. *J. Biol. Chem.* 1997 Jul 11;272(28):17390-4.

[234] Tippett PS, Neet KE. Specific inhibition of glucokinase by long chain acyl coenzymes A below the critical micelle concentration. *J. Biol. Chem.* 1982 Nov 10;257(21):12839-45.

[235] Bai FL, Yamano M, Shiotani Y, Emson PC, Smith AD, Powell JF, et al. An arcuato-paraventricular and -dorsomedial hypothalamic neuropeptide Y-containing system which lacks noradrenaline in the rat. *Brain Res.* 1985 Apr 1;331(1):172-5.

[236] Brady LS, Smith MA, Gold PW, Herkenham M. Altered expression of hypothalamic neuropeptide mRNAs in food-restricted and food-deprived rats. *Neuroendocrinology.* 1990 Nov;52(5):441-7.

[237] Akabayashi A, Zaia CT, Silva I, Chae HJ, Leibowitz SF. Neuropeptide Y in the arcuate nucleus is modulated by alterations in glucose utilization. *Brain Res.* 1993 Sep 10;621(2):343-8.

[238] Bagnol D, Lu XY, Kaelin CB, Day HE, Ollmann M, Gantz I, et al. Anatomy of an endogenous antagonist: relationship between Agouti-related protein and proopiomelanocortin in brain. *J. Neurosci.* 1999 Sep 15;19(18):RC26.

[239] Lu H, Buison A, Jen KC, Dunbar JC. Leptin resistance in obesity is characterized by decreased sensitivity to proopiomelanocortin products. *Peptides.* 2000 Oct;21(10):1479-85.

[240] Chen AS, Metzger JM, Trumbauer ME, Guan XM, Yu H, Frazier EG, et al. Role of the melanocortin-4 receptor in metabolic rate and food intake in mice. *Transgenic Res.* 2000 Apr;9(2):145-54.

[241] Baskin DG, Breininger JF, Schwartz MW. Leptin receptor mRNA identifies a subpopulation of neuropeptide Y neurons activated by fasting in rat hypothalamus. *Diabetes.* 1999 Apr;48(4):828-33.

[242] Baker RA, Herkenham M, Brady LS. Effects of long-term treatment with antidepressant drugs on proopiomelanocortin and neuropeptide Y mRNA expression in the hypothalamic arcuate nucleus of rats. *J. Neuroendocrinol.* 1996 May;8(5):337-43.

[243] Kow LM, Pfaff DW. Vasopressin excites ventromedial hypothalamic glucose-responsive neurons *in vitro*. *Physiol. Behav.* 1986;37(1):153-8.

[244] Kai Y, Oomura Y, Shimizu N. Responses of rat lateral hypothalamic neuron activity to dorsal raphe nuclei stimulation. *J. Neurophysiol.* 1988 Aug;60(2):524-35.

[245] Nishino H, Oomura Y, Karadi Z, Lenard L, Kai Y, Fukuda A, et al. Internal and external information processing by lateral hypothalamic glucose-sensitive and insensitive neurons during bar press feeding in the monkey. *Brain Res. Bull.* 1988 Jun;20(6):839-45.

Index